COURTNEY BLACK

Happier, Healthier, Tastier!

100 Healthy & Delicious Recipes

Thorsons
An imprint of HarperCollins*Publishers*
1 London Bridge Street
London SE1 9GF

www.harpercollins.co.uk

HarperCollins*Publishers*
1st Floor, Watermarque Building, Ringsend Road
Dublin 4, Ireland

First published by Thorsons 2022

10 9 8 7 6 5 4 3 2 1

Text © Courtney Black 2022
Photography © Anna Fowler 2022
Food photography © Andrew Burton and Sam
Folan 2022

Courtney Black asserts the moral right
to be identified as the author of this work

Contributing Writers: Oliver Downey (food)
Stylist: Georgie Gray
Hair: Jack Luckhurst
Make-up: Roqa Beauty
Food Stylist: Pippa Leon
Food Stylist's assistants: Simone Shagam
and Sian Williams
Prop Stylist: Lauren Miller

A catalogue record of this book is
available from the British Library

ISBN 978-0-00-852757-0

Printed and bound by GPS

MIX
Paper from
responsible sources
FSC™ C007454

FSC
www.fsc.org

This book is produced from independently certified FSC™ paper
to ensure responsible forest management.

For more information visit: www.harpercollins.co.uk/green

COURTNEY BLACK

Happier, Healthier, Tastier!

100 Healthy & Delicious Recipes

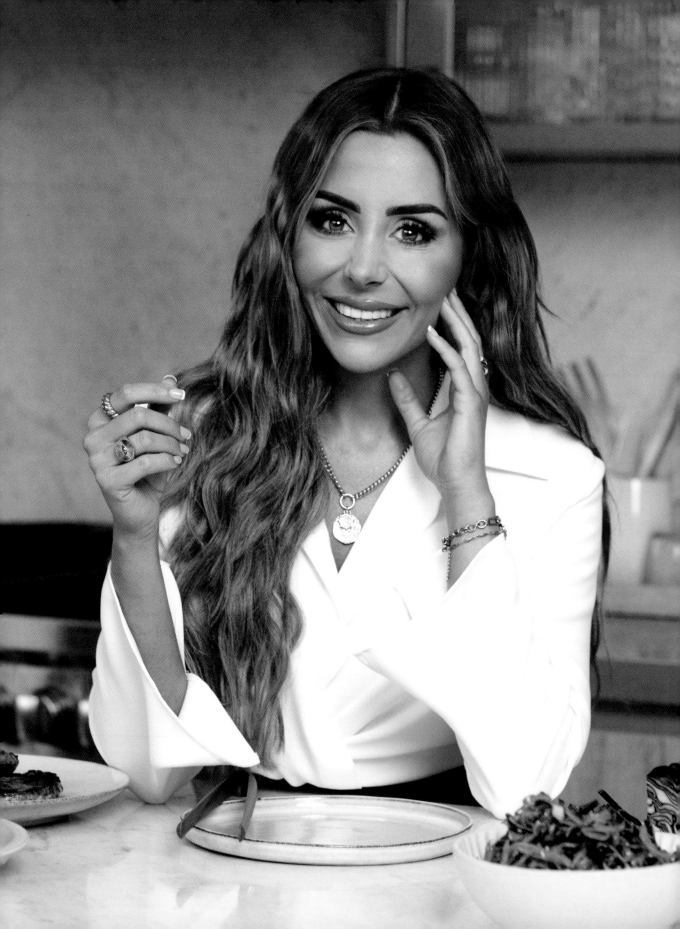

Contents

Introduction

Welcome to my fabulous new cookbook, which is packed with tasty new recipes for every season and occasion. I've got you covered with ideas for everything from breakfast on-the-go to weekend brunches, packed lunches, fakeaway suppers and entertaining your family and friends. As always, the recipes are all healthy and nutritious and, at under 600 calories max per serving, you can continue to enjoy all your favourite foods without missing out on flavour or worrying about what you're eating.

Enjoy your cooking

I want you to enjoy cooking – it's so satisfying and relaxing, and it makes you more aware of what you're putting into your body. My recipes are easy to follow, to prep and make, and you don't have to spend hours in the kitchen slaving over a hot stove. Nor do you need specialist skills; even if you're a complete novice when it comes to cooking from scratch, you'll quickly get the hang of it and be dishing up amazing meals in no time at all. Cooking is such an important part of building and enhancing a positive relationship with food. And to help you, I've come up with some useful guidelines and practical tips to make it even easier.

Courtney x

Happier, Healthier, Tastier!

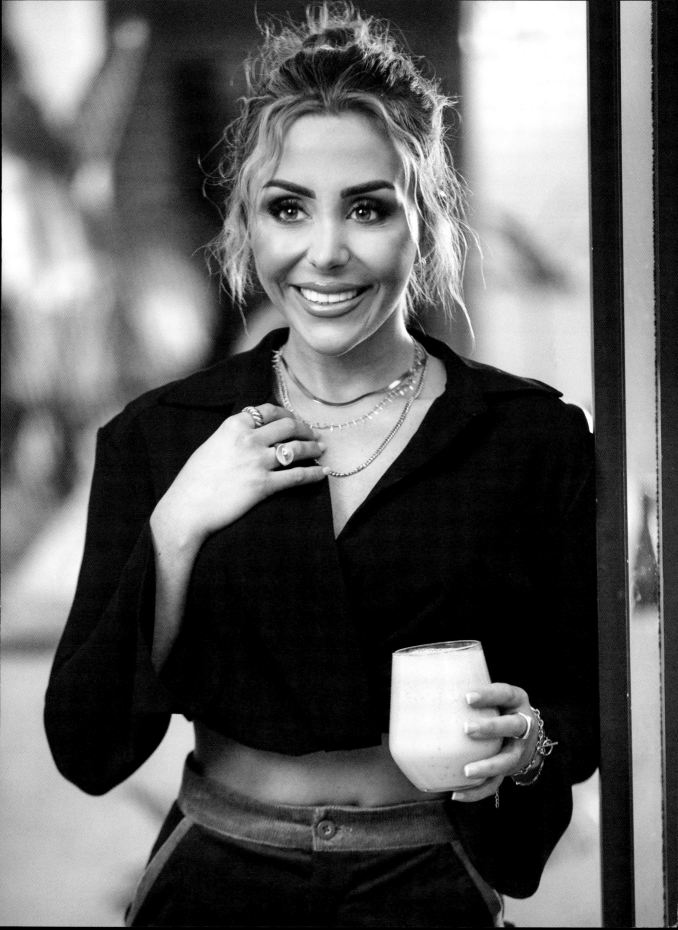

Essential kitchen equipment

Start by investing in some basic equipment and gadgets. They'll take the hard work out of so many tasks, from beating eggs and whisking up smoothies to puréeing vegetable soups and baking cakes. They'll speed up your prepping and help you to cook in a healthier and hassle-free way. Here's a suggested list to get you started:

Pots, pans and dishes

A small non-stick frying pan for omelettes, frittatas, quesadillas, etc.

A large non-stick frying pan for fish, chicken, steaks, cooked breakfasts, etc.

A small non-stick saucepan for making sauces, porridge, etc.

A few saucepans in different sizes with lids

A casserole dish and some ovenproof baking dishes

Roasting pans and baking trays

Cake tins (in different shapes and sizes), muffin tins and wire cooling racks

A wok (non-stick or seasoned) for stir-frying – although you can also use a deep frying pan

A ridged grill/griddle pan for meat, chicken, fish, seafood, vegetables, tofu and halloumi

Basic utensils

Wooden spoons, spatulas, slices

A good set of kitchen knives – different sizes and blades – plus a knife sharpener

Graters for vegetables and cheese, etc.

A balloon whisk

A colander and sieve

A measuring jug and scales, plus a set of measuring spoons

A rolling pin and pastry brush

Mixing bowls in different sizes

A potato masher

Metal or wooden skewers

Kitchen tongs

Speed peeler

Mason (Kilner) jars

Electrical equipment

An immersible hand blender

A food chopper, goblet blender or food processor

A hand-held electric whisk or food mixer

Special buys

If you're loving your cooking and feeling adventurous, how about splashing out on one of the following:

A waffle iron
Cookie rings and cutters
Piping bags and nozzles
A microwave
A barbecue

Happier, Healthier, Tastier!

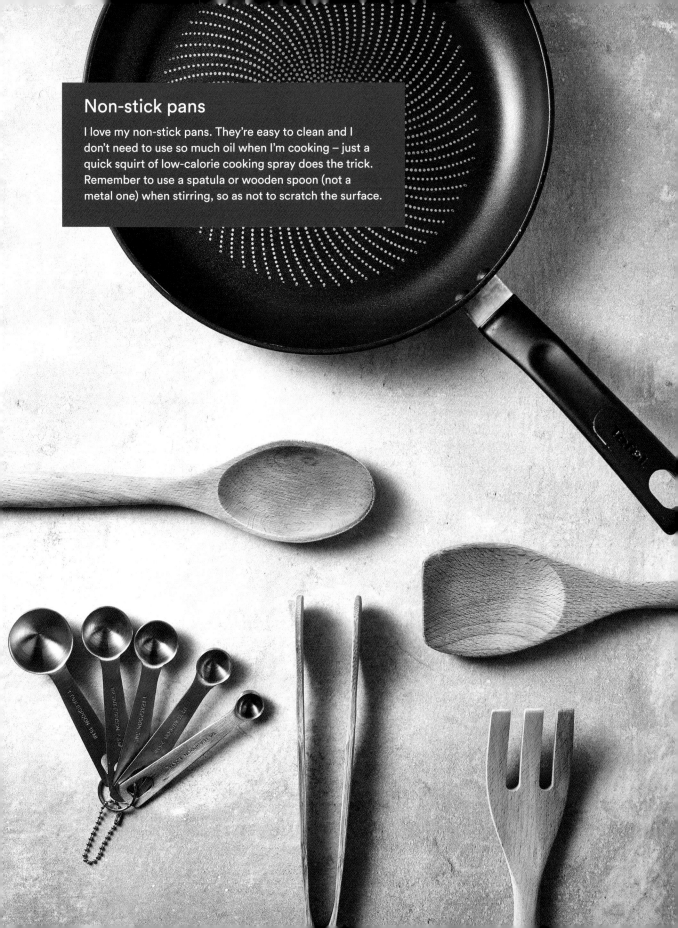

Non-stick pans

I love my non-stick pans. They're easy to clean and I don't need to use so much oil when I'm cooking – just a quick squirt of low-calorie cooking spray does the trick. Remember to use a spatula or wooden spoon (not a metal one) when stirring, so as not to scratch the surface.

Stock up on the basics

If you keep your store cupboard, fridge and freezer well stocked with essential foods, you'll never have an excuse not to cook a healthy meal. And with plenty of foods to hand, you won't have to make daily shopping trips to the supermarket for ready meals or order expensive takeaways. So be prepared and take a leaf out of my book with these suggestions for stocking up.

Store cupboard

CONDIMENTS AND FLAVOURINGS

Sea salt

Black pepper

Ground spices: cumin, curry powder, garam masala, smoked paprika, turmeric

Seasonings: Cajun, fajita, peri peri

Chilli: chilli flakes, chilli paste, chilli powder

Mustard: Dijon, honey, English

Stocks: stock cubes, bouillon powder, stock pots

Vinegar: balsamic, cider, wine

SAUCES

Soy sauce: dark and light

Teriyaki/tamari sauce

Fish sauce (nam pla)

Hoisin sauce

Hot sauce: sweet chilli, sriracha, harissa

Pesto: green/red

COOKING OILS

Olive oil

Low-calorie cooking spray

PASTA, GRAINS AND PULSES

Pasta shapes

Orzo

Spaghetti

Rolled oats

Rice: basmati, brown, risotto (Arborio)

Rice noodles

Red lentils

Cornflakes

CANS AND JARS

Light coconut milk

Beans: black, butter beans, cannellini

Chopped tomatoes

Chickpeas

Tomato purée

Tuna in brine or water

Passata

Black olives

Roasted peppers

Light mayo

BAKING

Plain flour

Self-raising flour

Baking powder

Bicarbonate of soda

Cornflour

Granulated sweetener

Maple syrup

Honey

Cocoa powder

Chocolate chips

Vanilla extract

Protein powder

Dried breadcrumbs

NUTS AND SEEDS

Nuts: flaked almonds, hazelnuts, roasted peanuts, walnuts

Nut butter: almond, peanut

Seeds: mixed, cumin, pumpkin, sesame

Happier, Healthier, Tastier!

Fridge and freezer

DAIRY AND VEGAN

Milk: skimmed, semi-skimmed, almond, oat

Reduced-fat spread

Yoghurt: low-fat, 0% fat, non-dairy (e.g. soya)

Reduced-fat cheese: Cheddar, feta, Mozzarella

Parmesan

Free-range eggs

Tofu

Quorn

FRUIT AND VEGETABLES

Fruit: lemons, limes

Vegetables: garlic, onions, green vegetables (e.g. broccoli), carrots

Salads: spring onions, salad leaves, tomatoes, peppers, cucumber

Fresh herbs: parsley, coriander, chives

Fresh spices: ginger, chillies, lemongrass

JARS

Curry paste

Coconut oil

FROZEN FOODS

Peas

Prawns

Chicken breasts

Minced beef

Tortillas and pita bread

Puff pastry

Healthy flavourings

Healthy, low-cal foods don't have to taste boring and bland. I use a variety of condiments, sauces, herbs and spices to add flavour, plus the finishing touches that transform my meals into something really delish. Here are some ideas to inspire you.

BASIC CONDIMENTS (SAVOURY AND SWEET)

Sea salt: choose from finely ground, coarse crystals and flakes

Pepper: choose from black, white or red/pink – black peppercorns are the most pungent of all

Balsamic vinegar: a syrupy, full-flavoured one is fabulous; drizzle over roasted vegetables, grilled chicken, tofu, salads and even strawberries!

Mustard: choose from Dijon, English, wholegrain and honey mustard; use sparingly in salad dressings, white sauces, marinades and glazes

Stock cubes and bouillon powder: choose from chicken, beef, fish, vegetable and porcini; use for flavouring soups, casseroles, stews, sauces, and cooking rice and grains

Oranges, lemons and limes: use the squeezed juice and/or grated zest to add a zingy, refreshing flavour to salad dressings, grilled seafood and chicken, Thai and Mexican dishes, cakes and desserts

Vanilla: choose from handy bottles of vanilla extract, dried vanilla pods and seeds; use to enhance cakes, cookies, desserts, ice creams, smoothies, shakes and hot drinks

SAUCES

Tomato ketchup: who doesn't love ketchup with burgers, sausages, grills, fries, etc.; choose

Happier, Healthier, Tastier!

The magic of garlic

One of the healthiest – and smelliest – flavourings of all. Aromatic and pungent, it will enhance and flavour even the most boring and bland foods. Use it fresh or in dried powder form, granules and salt. You can even grow your own garlic chives in a flowerpot.

from hot ketchup and reduced-sugar

Soy, tamari, teriyaki and Thai fish sauces: use these salty, aromatic sauces in marinades, stir-fries, gravies, casseroles, curries, dips and Asian salad dressings

Hot sauces: choose from sweet chilli, Tabasco, sriracha, harissa and a host of Mexican and West Indian hot chilli sauces – add to salad dressings, marinades, stir-fries, soups, casseroles, etc.; Caution: use Tabasco and harissa (both are fiery hot) and sweet chilli (high in sugar) sparingly

Worcestershire sauce: add a few drops to soups, pie fillings, casseroles and stews for a more piquant flavour

Pesto: just a teaspoon of green or red pesto can enhance a salad dressing, a sandwich filling or some mayo; drizzle over grilled vegetables and chicken, soups and stews

HERBS (FRESH AND DRIED)

Basil: use fresh in tomato salads and pasta dishes or to make pesto; add a pinch of dried basil to pasta sauces, soups and tomato-cased dishes

Bay leaves: use fresh or dried to add an aromatic touch to sauces (especially white sauce), soups and casseroles; tie them into a little bundle with sprigs of fresh parsley and thyme to make a bouquet garni for flavouring a stew

Chives: fresh chives add a delicious oniony flavour to salads, dressings and stir-fries; sprinkle them over soup, baked potatoes and grilled food just before serving

Coriander: love it or hate it, fresh coriander is the go-to herb for Mexican and Asian food; try chopping it into mayo, spicy dressings and tomato salsa

Dill: delicately flavoured and feathery, dill is used in lots of Greek and Middle Eastern dishes; it's great for flavouring fish, in tzatziki and white sauces or stirred into yoghurt or mayo

Fennel: the fresh, feathery fronds and the dried seeds have a mild aniseed taste that goes well with fish; use in salads, mayo and for flavouring dips

Mint: available fresh or dried, as mint sauce or jelly; peppermint has the classic menthol taste, but you can buy fresh mint in many guises, including spearmint, apple mint and pineapple mint – use it for flavouring lamb, tabbouleh, tzatziki and many Middle Eastern dishes

Oregano: strongly flavoured; use with lamb, smoky grilled aubergine and in tomato sauces and salads

Parsley: who doesn't use this finely chopped to add a green garnish or finishing touch to almost anything; choose between curly and flat-leaf

Rosemary: this bittersweet, intensely flavoured herb is great for roasted vegetables, meats and chicken; use the woody stems (after stripping the leaves) as natural kebab skewers, and add the tiny blue flowers to a loaf-cake mixture or salad

Happier, Healthier, Tastier!

Sage: use in stuffings for chicken and lamb, in soups and sauces, to flavour chicken breasts wrapped in parma ham and fried in oil

Thyme: its tiny leaves add a slightly sweet taste to stuffings, soups, stews, roast and grilled meats and even cakes

SPICES (FRESH AND DRIED)

Cayenne: dust this fiery red powder over grilled meat and fish, gyros and vegetables gratins, especially cauliflower cheese, or add to curries

Chilli: use fresh, ground, crushed into flakes or made into a paste; be careful when handling fresh chillies as the hot ones (for example, bird's eye, Thai and Jamaican Bonnet) are very fiery and can make your eyes sting if you rub them after handling – add to curries, sauces, chili con carne, vegetable chilli, fresh salsa, Mexican, Thai, Indian and Asian food, salad dressings, savoury sprinkles and even chocolate cakes and desserts, if you want to give them a kick (and always use sparingly and taste as you go along – you can add more heat, but you can't take it away!)

Cinnamon: available as powder or sticks, this warming spice can be added to curries, soups, rice dishes, desserts, cakes, cookies, smoothies and hot chocolate and coffee drinks

Cumin: with its sweet nutty and earthy flavour, ground cumin or cumin seeds are a feature of many Middle Eastern and North African dishes; use in curries, root vegetable soup, couscous and baking

Ginger: available fresh or in powdered form, ginger is sweet, spicy and very pungent; you can grate, crush or chop the peeled fresh root and use it to flavour stir-fries, curries, soups, smoothies and juices; use the dried version in cakes, cookies and desserts or curries

Nutmeg: add some grated nutmeg to a white sauce, rice pudding, custard or a creamy dessert – or use with other spices to flavour curries

Paprika: use the sweet, hot and smoked varieties; sprinkle over gyros, souvlaki, baked dishes, gratins and fried eggs, add to soups, baked sweet potatoes and spicy mayo or use it smoked in Spanish tortillas

OTHER SPICES

Have fun cooking with ground allspice, cardamom, coriander, saffron, star anise and turmeric. They all add their own distinctive flavour to so many dishes, sweet and savoury. And they're all low in calories, fat, carbs and really healthy. And don't forget – if all else fails, you can always try a pinch of curry powder or garam masala if they seem appropriate!

Cheat with sweet

Instead of using sugar or honey as a sweetener for porridge, overnight oats, desserts and cookies, substitute chopped fresh fruit, puréed and stewed fruit (especially apples, peaches and apricots) or dried fruit, such as raisins, sultanas, dates and figs. They are high in nutrients, especially vitamins, fibre and essential minerals, and contain natural fructose. Or add some freshly squeezed orange juice.

Happier, Healthier, Tastier!

Let's celebrate!

When you're feeling fitter, healthier and happier, what could be better than to treat yourself to a special meal and celebrate – or simply enjoy a good meal with family or friends? At the end of this book, you'll find some great menus for entertaining at home. There's no need to eat out when you can cook up, say, your own Japanese meal, Turkish meze or Spanish fiesta. And if you fancy something traditional, I've got some delicious roast dinners, too. There's a BBQ feast for warm summer days or a chippie night in with your feet up in front of the TV, watching a good movie.

All the recipes are easy to make and you can prepare a lot of the food ahead to make healthy entertaining effortless and more fun – plus, if you do the prep in advance, you can relax with your guests with a glass of vino. Go on! You deserve it.

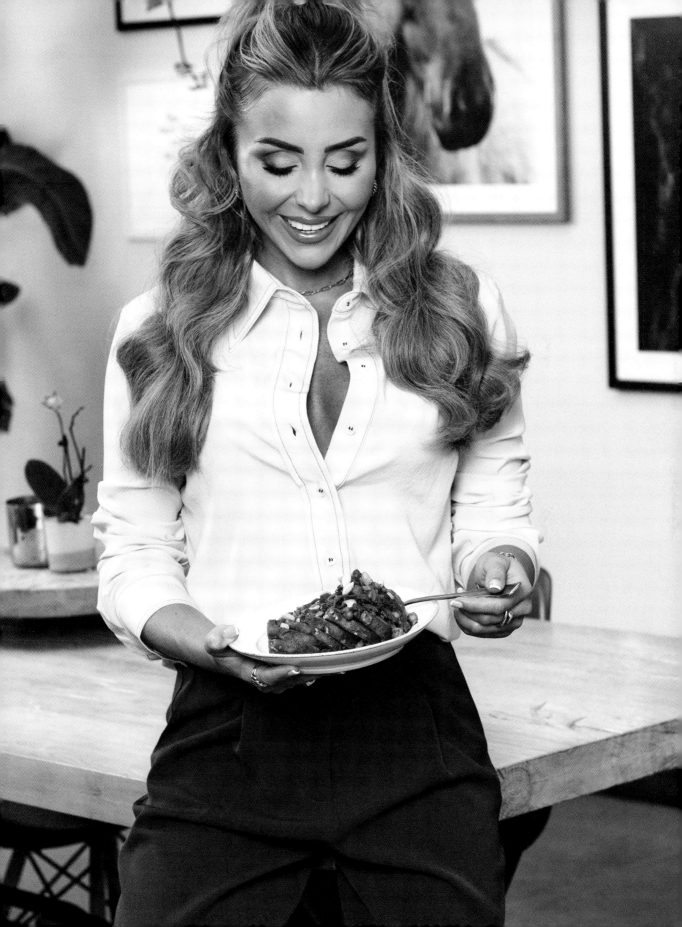

Meal Plans

Meal planning and menus

In the following pages you'll find so many delicious recipes for quick, tasty and nutritious meals, many of which will become your new go-to dishes. If you're always busy and rushing around like me, you probably don't have a lot of time to think about what you're going to eat and cook each day. However, by planning ahead and doing one big weekly shop you can get on with your life and focus on the important things – like making time to work out and chillax. With that in mind, here are some meal planners to inspire you.

Just take a few minutes to sit down and plan your menus, working around your diary and the recipes in this book, then make a shopping list and go for it. You can look forward to the week ahead with excitement and confidence, knowing that everything is under control and there won't be any boring meals on the menu!

General week planner

	MONDAY	TUESDAY	WEDNESDAY	THURSDAY	FRIDAY
BREAKFAST	SRIRACHA SMASHED EGGS (SEE PAGE 30)	SALMON AND LEEK FRITTATA (SEE PAGE 46)	PROTEIN BREAKFAST TACO WRAPS (SEE PAGE 40)	INDIAN BREAKFAST NAAN (SEE PAGE 47)	FULL ENGLISH BREAKFAST WRAP (SEE PAGE 50)
LUNCH	BOLOGNESE RISOTTO (SEE PAGE 131)	MASON-JAR PASTA SALAD (SEE PAGE 124)	CHEESE AND ONION PASTIES (SEE PAGE 118)	THAI CHICKEN BURGER (SEE PAGE 97)	LOADED HOT DOGS (SEE PAGE 111)
DINNER	TANDOORI SALMON BURGER (SEE PAGE 119)	FISH-FILLET BURGER (SEE PAGE 105)	BEEF PANANG CURRY (SEE PAGE 94)	MELT-IN-THE-MIDDLE FISHCAKES (SEE PAGE 112)	CHINESE CHAR SIU PORK (SEE PAGE 108)
DESSERT	RHUBARB AND APPLE CRUMBLES (SEE PAGE 230)	BAKED CUSTARD TARTS (SEE PAGE 220)	JAFFA CAKES (SEE PAGE 215)	BAKED CHURROS (SEE PAGE 216)	LEMON DRIZZLE CAKE (SEE PAGE 209)

Happier, Healthier, Tastier!

High-protein day planner 1

	DAY 1	DAY 2
BREAKFAST	PROTEIN BREAKFAST TACO WRAPS (SEE PAGE 40)	CHEESY BACON AND EGG BAGEL (SEE PAGE 31)
LUNCH	GREEK TURKEY BURGERS (SEE PAGE 64)	CHICKEN AND AVOCADO BURRITOS (SEE PAGE 144)
DINNER	CRISPY PORK SOUVLAKI (SEE PAGE 106)	CRISPY HALLOUMI FAJITAS (SEE PAGE 115)
DESSERT	OREO BROWNIES (SEE PAGE 226)	BISCOFF CHEESECAKE (SEE PAGE 211)

High-protein day planner 2

	DAY 1	DAY 2
BREAKFAST	BACON-STUFFED MUSHROOMS (SEE PAGE 28)	SAVOURY PROTEIN WAFFLES (SEE PAGE 49)
LUNCH	CHICKEN AND CHORIZO RICE (SEE PAGE 145)	CHILI CON PASTA BAKE (SEE PAGE 136)
DINNER	TANDOORI SALMON BURGER (SEE PAGE 119)	SUNRISE BURGER (SEE PAGE 98)
DESSERT	RHUBARB AND APPLE CRUMBLES (SEE PAGE 230)	SALTED PEANUT CHOCOLATE BARS (SEE PAGE 219)

Happier, Healthier, Tastier!

Rainy-day planner

BREAKFAST	LUNCH	DINNER	DESSERT
HOT CROSS BUNS (SEE PAGE 41)	NOURISHING ORZO SOUP (SEE PAGE 153)	QUICK CHORIZO AND RED PEPPER STEW (SEE PAGE 79)	BAKED CUSTARD TARTS (SEE PAGE 220)

Veggie/vegan weekly planner

	MONDAY	TUESDAY	WEDNESDAY	THURSDAY	FRIDAY
BREAKFAST	DOUBLE CHOCOLATE GRANOLA (SEE PAGE 44)	SAVOURY PROTEIN WAFFLES (SEE PAGE 49)	COCONUT AND CHIA BREAKFAST COOKIES (SEE PAGE 34)	STICKY TOFFEE BAKED OATS (SEE PAGE 38)	EASY HOMEMADE CRUMPETS (SEE PAGE 37)
LUNCH	TANDOORI LOADED SWEET POTATOES (VEGAN) (SEE PAGE 150)	STICKY AUBERGINE NOODLES (VEGAN) (SEE PAGE 168)	CHEESY 'SAUSAGE' ROLLS (SEE PAGE 164)	KOREAN BBQ JACKFRUIT RICE BOWL (VEGAN) (SEE PAGE 157)	NOURISHING ORZO SOUP (VEGAN) (SEE PAGE 153)
DINNER	ONE-POT GREEK ORZO (SEE PAGE 166)	EASY RED LENTIL DHAL (VEGAN) (SEE PAGE 159)	TOFU PAD THAI (VEGAN) (SEE PAGE 163)	ROASTED VEGETABLE PAELLA (SEE PAGE 160)	SPICY CAULIFLOWER STEAKS (VEGAN) (SEE PAGE 167)
DESSERT	FUDGE BROWNIES (VEGAN) (SEE PAGE 212)	SALTED PEANUT CHOCOLATE BARS (VEGAN) (SEE PAGE 219)	RHUBARB AND APPLE CRUMBLES (SEE PAGE 230)	MINI MILLIONAIRE SHORTBREADS (SEE PAGE 210)	BAKED CUSTARD TARTS (SEE PAGE 220)

Happier, Healthier, Tastier!

Breakfast & Brunch

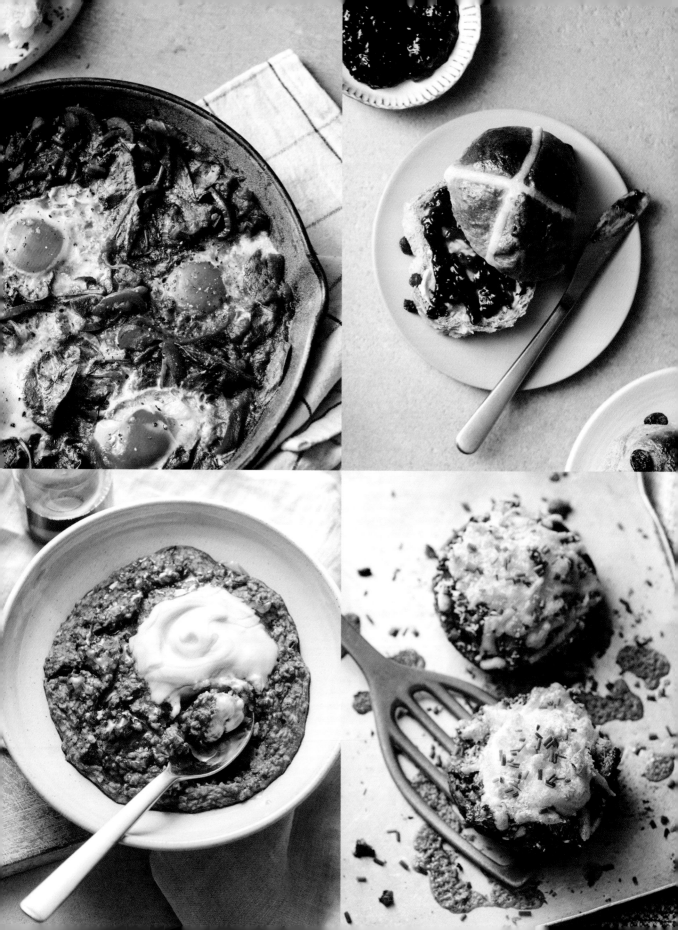

Maple Bacon Pancakes
Bacon-stuffed Mushrooms
Sriracha Smashed Eggs
Cheesy Bacon and Egg Bagel
Chorizo and Spinach Baked Eggs
Coconut and Chia Breakfast Cookies
Easy Homemade Crumpets
Sticky Toffee Baked Oats
Breakfast Breakfast Taco Wraps
Hot Cross Buns
Double Chocolate Granola
Salmon and Leek Frittata
Indian Breakfast Naan
Savoury Protein Waffles
Full English Breakfast Wrap

Maple Bacon Pancakes

Per serving:

Carbs: 41.5g

Calories: 344

Fat: 9.9g

Protein: 18.7g

Who would have thought that pancakes are so easy to make? They are the perfect weekend breakfast or brunch for all the family and taste as good as they look. You can even make the batter in advance and store it in the fridge overnight.

SERVES 4

8 rashers of smoked streaky
  bacon
185g plain flour
35g vanilla protein powder
2½ tsp baking powder
Pinch of salt
1 large egg, beaten
200ml semi-skimmed milk
Low-calorie cooking spray
2 tbsp maple syrup, plus extra
  for drizzling (optional)

1. Preheat the oven to 200°C/180°C Fan/Gas 6 and line a baking tray with non-stick baking paper.
2. Lay your bacon rashers out evenly on the tray and bake in the oven for 15–20 minutes, until crispy.
3. Meanwhile, combine the flour, protein power, baking powder and salt in a mixing bowl, then whisk in the beaten egg and half the milk, until the mixture is lump-free.
4. Gradually add the rest of the milk and the 2 tablespoons of maple syrup, whisking, until the batter is runny, but not too thin.
5. Heat a non-stick frying pan over a medium heat and lightly grease with low-calorie cooking spray.
6. Add 2 tablespoons of batter per pancake to the pan (it should make about 8 pancakes).
7. Once little bubbles form on the surface of the pancakes, slide a spatula underneath and flip. Repeat with the remaining batter.
8. Serve with the crispy bacon and a drizzle of maple syrup, if desired.

Happier, Healthier, Tastier!

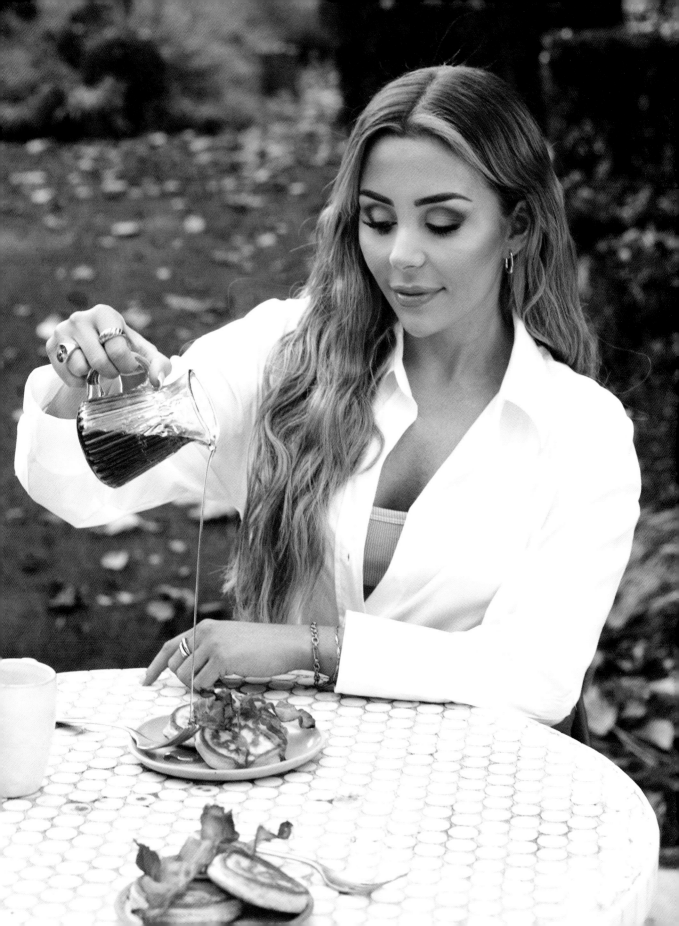

Bacon-stuffed Mushrooms

Per serving:

Carbs: 14.4g

Calories: 379

Fat: 13.1g

Protein: 53.5g

Why not shake up your breakfast with these delicious cheesy-topped mushrooms? They're so easy to make and ready to eat in just over fifteen minutes. And even better, they're low-carb, low-fat and high in protein. What's not to like?

SERVES 1

2 portobello (or flat field) mushrooms, stalks removed
Low-calorie cooking spray
155g smoked lean bacon, diced
½ small onion, finely chopped
½ garlic clove, finely grated
30g 50 per cent reduced-fat Cheddar, grated
2 tsp dried breadcrumbs
1 tsp chopped chives
Worcestershire sauce, for drizzling (optional)
Freshly ground black pepper

1. Preheat the oven to 220°C/200°C Fan/Gas 7.
2. Flip your mushrooms over so the holes are face-down, place on a baking tray and bake in the oven for 5 minutes.
3. Meanwhile, heat a non-stick frying pan over a medium–high heat and spray with low-calorie cooking spray. Add the diced bacon and fry for 3–5 minutes, until crisp.
4. Reduce the heat slightly, add the onion and garlic and fry for a further 2–3 minutes, until softened. Season everything with black pepper.
5. Remove the mushrooms from the oven and carefully flip over. Divide the bacon, onion and garlic mixture to fill each mushroom.
6. Sprinkle the cheese over each mushroom, followed by the breadcrumbs. Bake the filled mushrooms in the oven for around 8–10 minutes, until the cheese has melted and is beginning to turn golden.
7. Serve, sprinkled with the chopped chives and a splash of Worcestershire sauce, if using.

Happier, Healthier, Tastier!

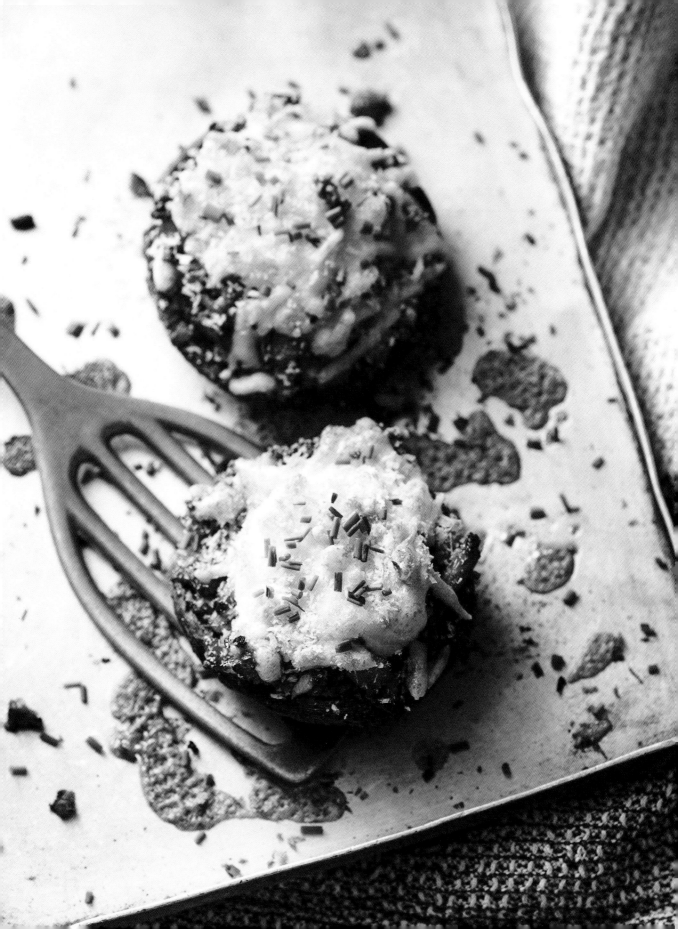

Sriracha Smashed Eggs (v)

Per serving:

Carbs: 26.5g

Calories: 350

Fat: 19.7g

Protein: 18g

If you love hot sauce as much as I do, you won't be able to resist these delicious smashed eggs on avocado toast. And they're so quick and easy that you can rustle them up in a few minutes before you leave home for work, college or the school run.

SERVES 1

2 large eggs
½ tsp sriracha sauce
1 tbsp low-fat soft cream cheese
1 slice of sourdough (or your preferred bread)
Squeeze of lime juice
¼ avocado, mashed
½ red chilli, deseeded and finely sliced
½ punnet fresh cress
2 tbsp fresh coriander, torn
1 tsp mixed seeds
Sea salt
Freshly ground black pepper

1. Boil a saucepan of water over a high heat, then set a timer for 7 minutes and carefully lower the eggs into the pan. Press go on the timer!
2. Meanwhile, mix the sriracha and low-fat cream cheese together, then season with some sea salt and black pepper.
3. Toast the bread and then spread with the creamy sriracha.
4. Mix the lime juice with the mashed avocado and spoon this over the top.
5. Remove your eggs from the pan with a slotted spoon and carefully peel them. Place them in a bowl and lightly mash them with a fork, then add on top of the avocado.
6. Top everything off with the red chilli, cress, fresh coriander and mixed seeds.

Happier, Healthier, Tastier!

Cheesy Bacon and Egg Bagel

Per serving:

Carbs: 29.1g

Calories: 587

Fat: 35.5g

Protein: 33.5g

Nothing beats a lightly toasted bagel. And my fried egg, bacon and avocado filling makes a tasty change from the usual smoked salmon and cream cheese. Make sure you use a thin bagel for this recipe as the larger, thicker ones can be surprisingly high in carbs and calories.

SERVES 1

2 rashers of smoked streaky bacon
1 tsp olive oil
1 egg
1 plain thin bagel, halved
¼ avocado, mashed
1 slice of reduced-fat mild cheese
1 tsp fresh chives, finely chopped
Sea salt
Freshly ground black pepper

1. Preheat the oven to 200°C/180°C Fan/Gas 6 and line a baking tray with non-stick baking paper.
2. Lay your bacon rashers out evenly on the tray and bake in the oven for 15–20 minutes, until crispy.
3. Meanwhile, heat the olive oil in a non-stick frying pan over a medium heat and, once hot, crack in the egg and fry for around 4–5 minutes, until the white is set but the yolk is still runny. Season with sea salt and black pepper and transfer to a piece of kitchen paper.
4. Lightly toast the bagel halves, until golden, then pile the mashed avocado, bacon, cheese slice, egg and a sprinkling of chives on to the bottom half.
5. Finish with the top half of the bagel and press down to allow the delicious yolk to run through.

Happier, Healthier, Tastier!

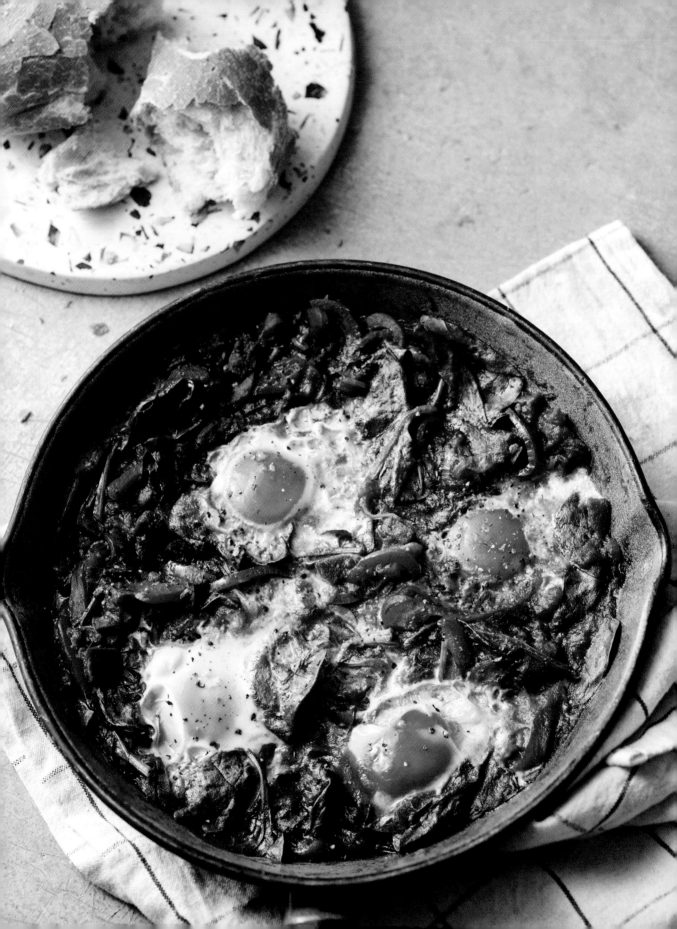

Chorizo and Spinach Baked Eggs

Per serving:

Carbs: 14.7g

Calories: 435

Fat: 28.6g

Protein: 18.3g

Add a touch of sunny Spain to your breakfast with some spicy chorizo and smoked paprika. They will transform simple baked eggs into something truly special. This also makes a delicious brunch or even a light lunch or supper, served with crusty bread.

SERVES 2

1 tsp olive oil
1 tsp chilli flakes
80g chorizo, cut into small
    cubes
1 red pepper, deseeded and
    finely sliced
1 red onion, finely sliced
3 garlic cloves, finely grated
1 tbsp smoked paprika
1 tbsp balsamic vinegar
1 × 400g tin chopped tomatoes
80g baby spinach
4 large eggs
Sea salt
Freshly ground black pepper

1. Heat the olive oil in a large non-stick frying pan (one that has a lid) over a medium heat and fry the chilli flakes, chorizo, red pepper and onion for about 5 minutes, until the chorizo has released its delicious golden oil and the onion and pepper are softening.
2. Add the garlic to the pan and fry for a further 3–4 minutes, stirring frequently.
3. Sprinkle in the smoked paprika and stir everything well. Fry for another minute.
4. Season well with sea salt and black pepper, then stir in the balsamic vinegar and chopped tomatoes, along with a splash of water.
5. Add the spinach, stir into the sauce and reduce the heat to low. Leave to bubble for 10 minutes – this will help to thicken the sauce and allow you to create holes for the eggs.
6. Using a wooden spoon, make four wells in the sauce and crack an egg into each one. Cover the frying pan with a lid and cook for around 8 minutes, until the eggs are just set. Serve with crusty bread.

Happier, Healthier, Tastier!

Coconut and Chia Breakfast Cookies ⓥ

Per cookie:

Carbs: 12g

Calories: 71

Fat: 2.4g

Protein: 1.6g

If you're in a hurry and don't have time for breakfast before leaving home, don't worry . . . just grab some of these yummy cookies and munch them on the go. You can batch bake them in advance and store them in an airtight container for up to three days.

MAKES 10
2 ripe bananas
80g rolled oats
25g desiccated coconut
1 tbsp chia seeds
1 tsp vanilla extract
½ tbsp maple syrup
A splash of milk (if needed)

1. Preheat the oven to 190°C/170°C Fan/Gas 5 and line a baking tray with non-stick baking paper.
2. In a bowl, mash the bananas, until smooth. Add the rest of the ingredients and mix together. If the mixture is a little too dry, add a tiny splash of milk (or plant alternative).
3. Roll the mixture into 10 equal balls and place on the prepared baking tray, flattening them a little with the palm of your hand.
4. Bake for 15–20 minutes, until lightly golden. Leave to cool and harden slightly before serving.

Happier, Healthier, Tastier!

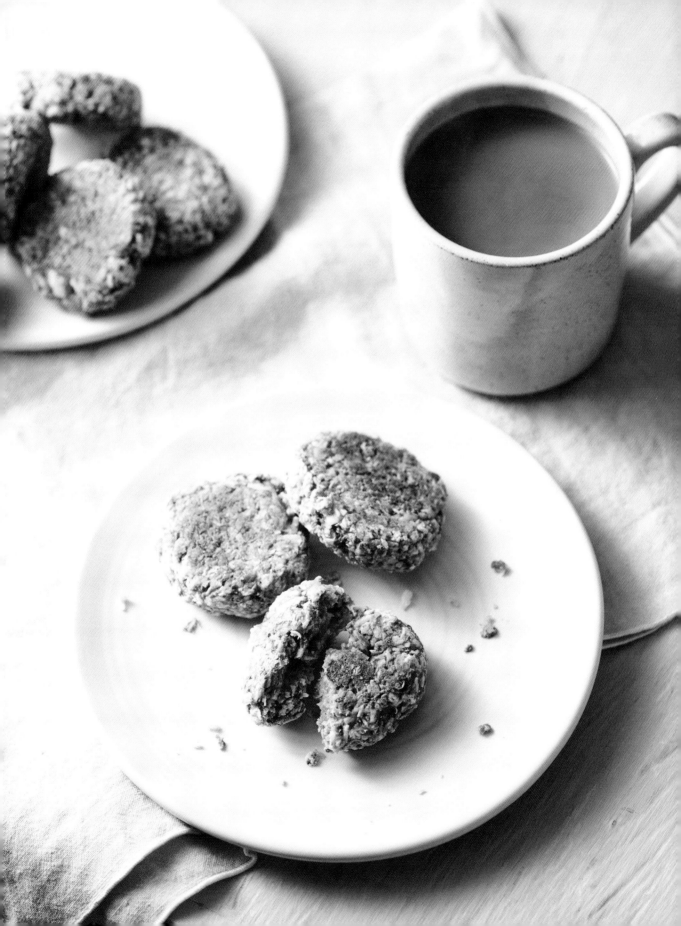

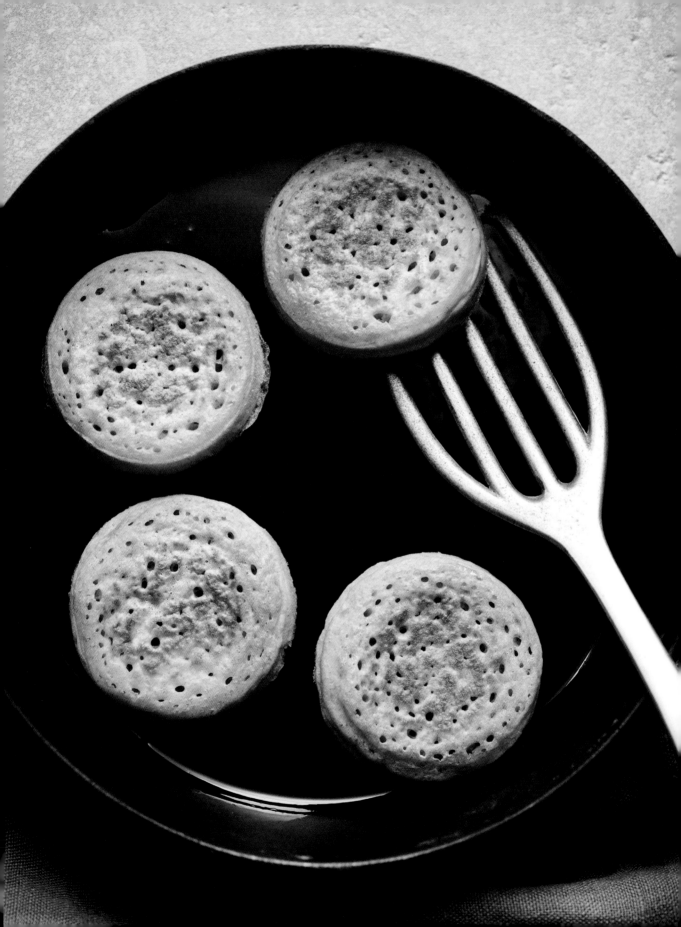

Easy Homemade Crumpets

Per crumpet:

Carbs: 17.8g

Calories: 102

Fat: 1.4g

Protein: 2.7g

It may sound like a bit off a faff, but making your own crumpets really is worth it. If you enjoy baking and have half an hour to spare, give it a go! They're so tasty and healthier than most of the crumpets on sale in supermarkets . . . and they're fun to make, too. Top with a poached egg or grilled mushrooms, some sliced tomato, smashed avocado or crispy bacon to make more of a meal.

MAKES 6
150g plain flour
½ tsp caster sugar (don't leave this out – it's important!)
1 tsp baking powder (or 1 × 5g sachet)
200ml warm water, plus 1 tbsp
1 tsp dried active yeast
1 tsp salt
Low-calorie cooking spray
1 tbsp low-fat spread (or butter)

1. In a large bowl, whisk the flour, sugar and baking powder with the 200ml warm water and salt for 2–3 minutes, until smooth.
2. In a small bowl, mix the tablespoon of warm water with the yeast to dissolve it.
3. Add the yeast and warm water to the larger bowl and whisk everything together, ensuring no lumps remain.
4. Cover the bowl with cling film and leave in a warm place for 30 minutes, until the surface looks bubbly.
5. Grease the insides of some crumpet-sized metal cookie rings/ cutters with low-calorie cooking spray.
6. Melt the low-fat spread in a non-stick frying pan over a medium heat. Pour some batter into the rings and fry for 1½ minutes, until you see bubbles on the surface.
7. Continue cooking for another minute, then reduce the heat to low and gently cook for a further 3–4 minutes, until the crumpets seem set and no new bubbles appear.
8. Remove the crumpets from the rings, flip them over and cook the tops for up to 1 minute.
9. These can be stored and popped in the toaster to reheat for the next few days!

Happier, Healthier, Tastier!

Sticky Toffee Baked Oats (v)

Per serving:

Carbs: 78.1g

Calories: 445

Fat: 6.4g

Protein: 14g

If you have a sweet tooth, this is sure to become one of your favourites. Oats are not only a good source of protein, but also low GI, helping to regulate your blood-sugar levels and releasing energy more slowly throughout the day – the perfect food if you're planning to work out or go for a run.

SERVES 1

40g rolled oats

35g ripe banana, mashed

1 tbsp zero-calorie maple syrup, plus 1 tsp for drizzling

150g low-fat toffee yoghurt

1 large egg white

½ tsp baking powder

1 tsp cocoa powder

2 pitted dates, finely chopped

1. Preheat the oven to 200°C/180°C Fan/Gas 6.
2. In a large bowl, mix together the oats, banana, the tablespoon of maple syrup, 120g of the toffee yoghurt, the egg white, baking powder, cocoa powder and dates.
3. Line a small roasting dish with non-stick baking paper, then pour in the mixture and bake in the oven for 35–40 minutes, until golden and cooked through.
4. Spoon over the remaining toffee yoghurt, drizzle with maple syrup and enjoy.

Happier, Healthier, Tastier!

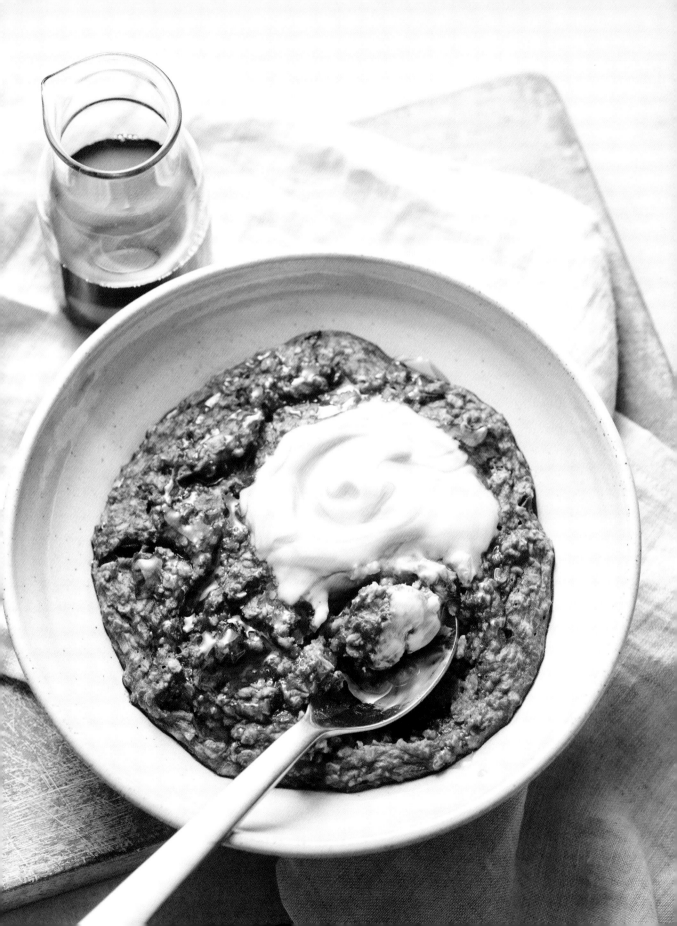

Protein Breakfast Taco Wraps

Per serving:

Carbs: 20.6g

Calories: 517

Fat: 42.5g

Protein: 58.3g

These mouthwateringly good wraps, oozing with melted cheese, are one of my all-time favourites! And they're perfect for a weekend brunch or a light lunch – just double the quantities if you have guests. Your kids will love them, too. Vegetarians can substitute Quorn mince for the beef.

MAKES 2

Low-calorie cooking spray
300g lean beef mince
1 tsp taco mix
4 large eggs, beaten
2 tortilla wraps
30g reduced-fat mozzarella, grated
30g reduced-fat Cheddar, grated
2 large handfuls of baby spinach
2 tbsp fat-free yoghurt
2 tsp chilli paste
Sea salt
Freshly ground black pepper

1. Heat a large non-stick frying pan over a medium heat and grease well with cooking spray. Fry the beef mince for 6–8 minutes, breaking up with a wooden spoon, until cooked through. Sprinkle in the taco mix and season well with sea salt and black pepper.
2. When your beef mince has been frying for 5 minutes, heat another smaller frying pan over a medium–high heat and grease with cooking spray. Pour in the beaten eggs and stir well. If your pan is hot enough, they should scramble within a couple of minutes.
3. Lay a tortilla wrap out and slice through from the middle to the edge directly in front of you.
4. Lay some beef mince in top left quarter of the wrap, then top the beef with some cheese. Place the egg in the top right quarter and a handful of spinach in the bottom right quarter.
5. With the slit side facing you vertically, lift the empty quarter (next to the slit), and fold it up so the beef and cheese are now covered. Then fold sideways on top of the egg and again, so that the egg is on top of the spinach.
6. Return the wrap to the pan to heat through for 30–60 seconds on each side, until the cheese has melted and the wrap is golden. Repeat with remaining wrap and fillings.
7. Mix together the fat-free yoghurt and chilli paste to make a dip for your tacos.

Happier, Healthier, Tastier!

Hot Cross Buns Ⓥ

I love these buns so much that I can happily bake them at any time of the year. They take a little time to make, but are so superior to shop-bought ones and well worth the effort. The sweet, spicy aroma wafts through the kitchen and throughout my home. Eat fresh and warm from the oven or split and toast them and enjoy with melting low-fat spread and fruity jam.

Per bun:

Carbs: 40g

Calories: 231

Fat: 4.7g

Protein: 7g

MAKES 12
50g butter
220ml semi-skimmed milk
450g strong white bread flour, plus extra for dusting
7g sachet of fast-action yeast
2 tbsp caster sugar
1 tsp ground cinnamon
2 tsp ground allspice
½ tsp ground nutmeg
1 tbsp granulated sweetener
1 tsp salt
150g raisins
2 large eggs, beaten
Low-calorie cooking spray
50g plain flour

1. Heat the butter in a small pan over a low heat, until completely melted. Transfer to a small bowl and set aside, then wipe out the pan and heat the milk over a low heat, until warm.
2. Sift the flour into a large bowl, then add the yeast, sugar, spices, sweetener and salt. Mix through the raisins.
3. Make a well with your hand in the dry ingredients and add the melted butter, warm milk and one of the eggs. Using a knife, bring the dry ingredients into the wet and then, when it gets too difficult, use your hands to combine everything into a dough.
4. Flour the work surface, then transfer the dough out of the bowl and knead with your hands, until smooth (this should take around 2–3 minutes).
5. Spray a large mixing bowl with cooking spray to grease it, then add the dough to the bowl. Cover with a tea towel and leave it in a warm place for up to 2 hours, until it has doubled in size.
6. Dust the work surface with flour, then add the dough and knead again for 30 seconds. Divide the dough into 12 equal amounts, then form each one into a hot-cross bun shape.
7. Spray a baking tray with low-calorie cooking spray, then add the buns, cover with cling film and leave, until they have again doubled in size.
8. Preheat the oven to 200°C/180°C Fan/Gas 6. Remove the cling film from the buns. Beat the other egg and brush it over the top of each bun.
9. Mix the plain flour with water in a small bowl – this should make a paste that you will be able to pipe onto the buns for the 'cross'. Add the paste to a piping bag and attach a small nozzle. Score a cross over the top of each one with a small knife, then pipe on the paste.
10. Bake the buns for around 20 minutes, until they have risen and turned golden.

Happier, Healthier, Tastier!

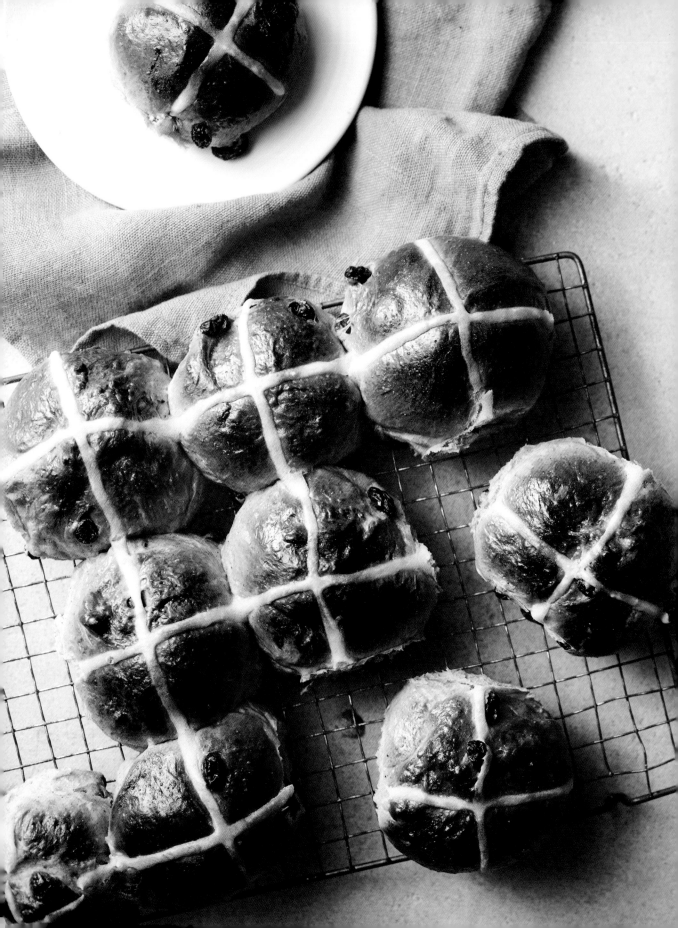

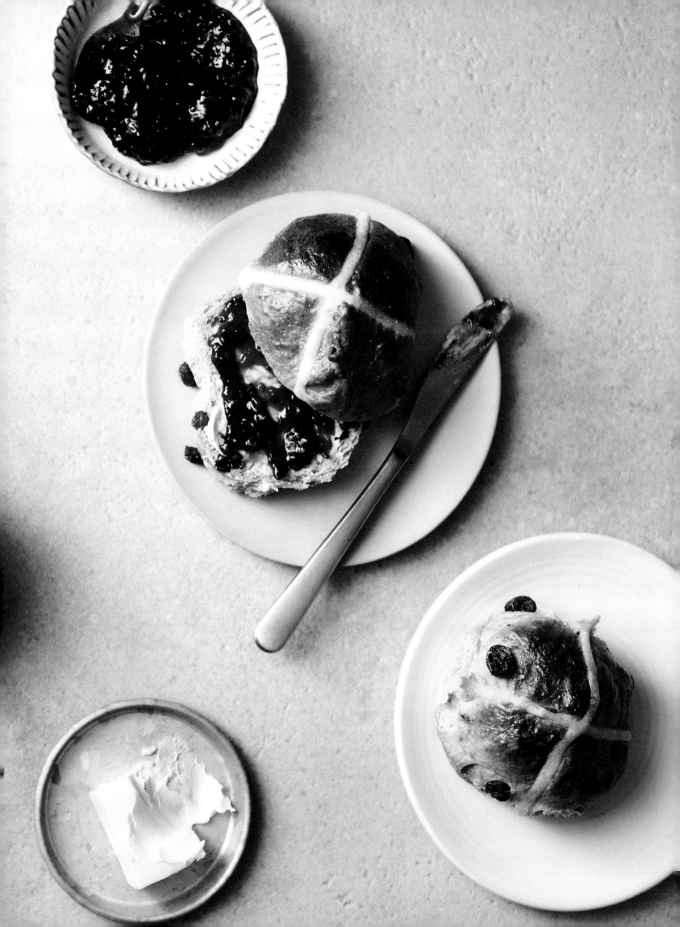

Double Chocolate Granola

Per serving:

Carbs: 31.8g

Calories: 308

Fat: 15.7g

Protein: 9.3g

This granola is as good as it gets, and so much tastier and more nutritious than many of the commercially produced ones in your local supermarket. Serve it with nut milk or Greek 0 per cent fat yoghurt and fresh, juicy berries for a quick and easy breakfast when you're in a hurry.

MAKES 15 SERVINGS

50g coconut oil, melted

1 tsp vanilla extract

60g maple syrup

400g rolled oats

35g vanilla or chocolate protein powder

2 tbsp cocoa powder

2 tsp ground cinnamon

½ tsp sea salt

50g pumpkin seeds

50g walnuts, roughly chopped

50g hazelnuts, roughly chopped

100g dried raisins

80g flaked almonds

100g milk (or dark) chocolate chips

1. Preheat the oven to 180°C/160°C Fan/Gas 4 and line two baking trays with non-stick baking paper.
2. In a large bowl, combine the melted coconut oil, vanilla extract and maple syrup.
3. Add the rolled oats, protein and cocoa powders, cinnamon, salt, pumpkin seeds, walnuts and hazelnuts, and stir well to ensure everything is well coated.
4. Arrange the granola over the prepared baking trays, ensuring it is more or less in an even layer, and bake in the oven for around 25–30 minutes, turning halfway through. It should be nice and golden all over.
5. Leave to cool, then transfer to a large bowl and stir through the raisins, flaked almonds and chocolate chips. Store in an airtight container or jar for up to 3 weeks.

Happier, Healthier, Tastier!

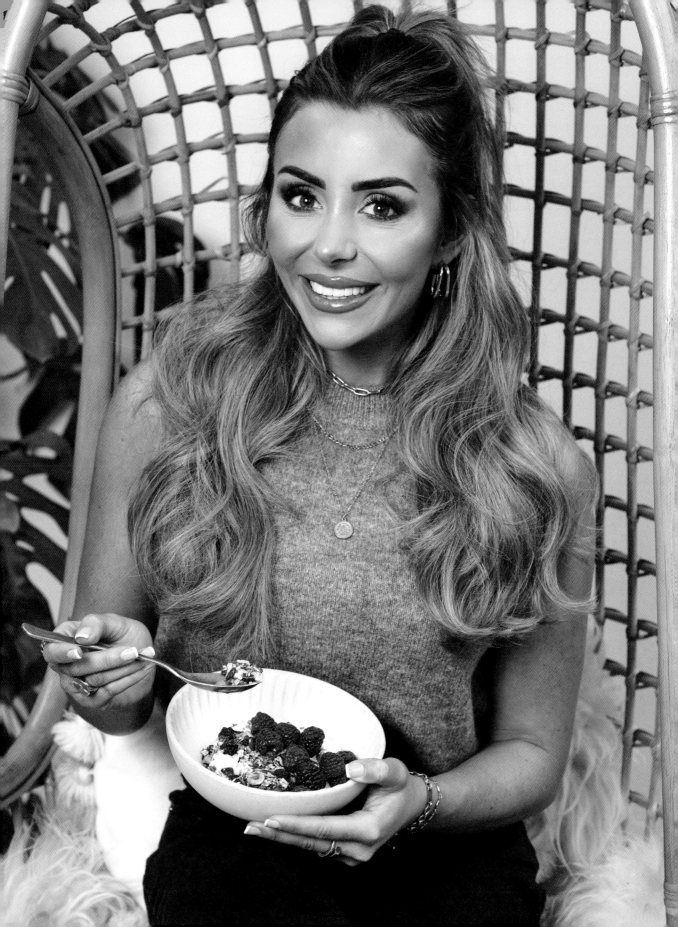

Salmon and Leek Frittata

Per serving:

Carbs: 14.4g

Calories: 536

Fat: 33.1g

Protein: 43.7g

When you wake up feeling peckish or need a protein boost to start the day, this is the perfect breakfast. The salmon, eggs and cheese are all packed with protein, as well as a jackpot of healthy vitamins and minerals. And it's great for weekend brunches, too.

SERVES 2

1 tsp olive oil
½ onion, finely sliced
1 leek, trimmed and very finely sliced
2 garlic cloves, finely grated
1 heaped tsp Dijon mustard
180g hot smoked salmon fillets, flaked into large chunks
6 eggs, beaten
40g reduced-fat Cheddar, grated
Freshly ground black pepper

1. Heat the olive oil in a non-stick, ovenproof frying pan over a medium heat and add the onion and leek. Fry for 3–5 minutes, until softened and slightly golden.
2. Add the garlic and fry for a further 2 minutes.
3. Stir through the Dijon mustard and flaked salmon, carefully stirring for a couple of minutes.
4. Add the beaten eggs to the pan and season with black pepper. Stir carefully to move the eggs around, ensuring the bottom of the pan is covered. Cook for 2–3 minutes, until nearly set.
5. Sprinkle over the cheese, then turn the grill to medium–high and pop the pan under the grill for 1–2 minutes, until the cheese is lightly golden and the egg is cooked through.

Happier, Healthier, Tastier!

Indian Breakfast Naan

Per serving:

Carbs: 33.3g

Calories: 386

Fat: 19.3g

Protein: 14.8g

I'm a great fan of Indian food and even eat it for breakfast. This delicious naan, loaded with aromatic herbs, seeds, fruity chutney, soothing yoghurt and crispy bacon, will get your taste buds tingling. Go on . . . try it for yourself and see how good it tastes.

SERVES 1

2 rashers of smoked streaky bacon
1 tbsp cumin seeds
1 tsp olive oil
1 large egg
1 small naan
1 tbsp fat-free yoghurt
1 tbsp mango chutney
1 tbsp fresh coriander, torn
Sea salt
Freshly ground black pepper

1. Preheat the oven to 200°C/180°C Fan/Gas 6 and line a baking tray with non-stick baking paper.
2. Lay the bacon rashers out evenly on the tray and bake in the oven for 15–20 minutes, until crispy.
3. Heat a non-stick frying pan over a medium heat and, once hot, lightly toast the cumin seeds for 2 minutes, until fragrant. Remove from the pan and set aside.
4. Keeping the pan on the heat, drizzle in the olive oil and, once hot, crack in the egg and fry for 4–5 minutes, until the white is set, but the yolk is still runny. Season with sea salt and black pepper and transfer to a piece of kitchen paper.
5. Cook the naan in the oven, according to the packet instructions – it should take 3–4 minutes. Remove the naan from the oven, spread with the yoghurt, then follow with the mango chutney.
6. Top with the fried egg, then the crispy bacon.
7. Sprinkle over the toasted cumin seeds and fresh coriander and season with sea salt and black pepper.

Happier, Healthier, Tastier!

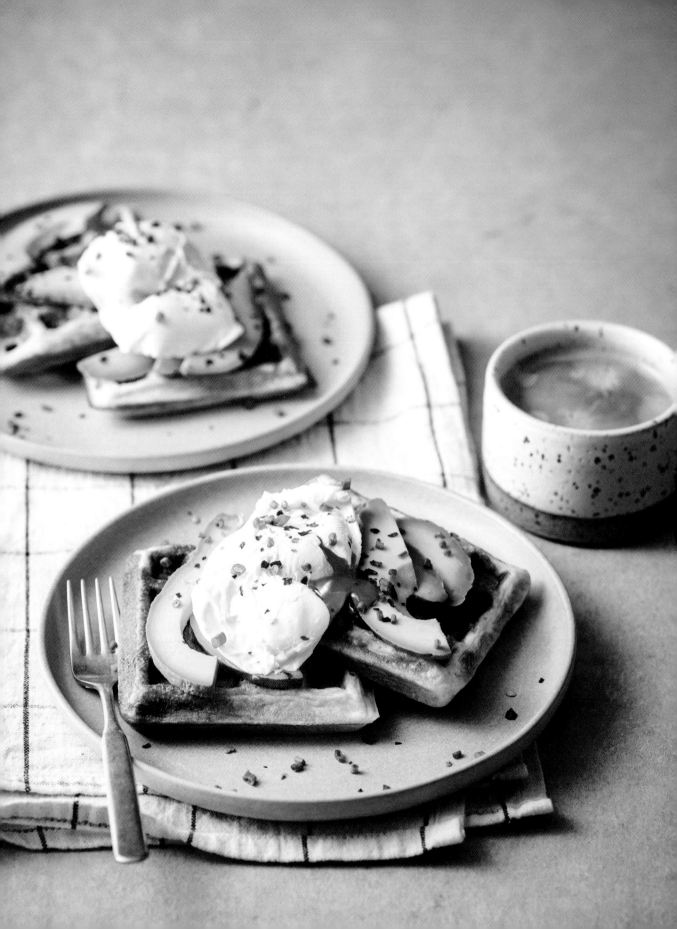

Savoury Protein Waffles ⓥ

Per serving:

Carbs: 23.6g

Calories: 414

Fat: 19.3g

Protein: 37.2g

You'll need a waffle machine for this recipe. They're not expensive and will be a good investment if you like waffles as much as I do. This fabulous savoury version is a delicious and healthier alternative to the more familiar sweet ones drenched in syrup. Try it and see for yourself!

SERVES 2

40g unflavoured protein powder
40g plain flour
20g Parmesan, grated
1 tsp baking powder
4 eggs, 2 beaten and 2 left whole for poaching
130ml skimmed milk
Low-calorie cooking spray
½ ripe avocado, sliced
1 tbsp fresh chives, finely sliced, to serve
½ tsp chilli flakes
Sea salt

1. Preheat a waffle iron to a high heat.
2. In a bowl, combine the protein powder, plain flour, Parmesan and baking powder and season well with sea salt. Add the beaten eggs and milk and whisk to a smooth batter.
3. Grease the waffle iron with low-calorie cooking spray and spoon part of the mixture on to the iron (depending on the machine, this may make two smaller waffles or one large at a time).
4. Add the remaining eggs to gently simmering water and poach to your liking (around 2–4 minutes, depending on how you like them).
5. Load each waffle with sliced avocado and a poached egg, then sprinkle over the chopped chives and chilli flakes.

Happier, Healthier, Tastier!

Full English Breakfast Wrap

Per serving:

Carbs: 27.6g

Calories: 561

Fat: 32.2g

Protein: 39g

If you enjoy a full English breakfast as much as I do, you'll love this. It's packed with nutritional goodness and delivers quite a protein punch to fuel your workout and keep you going throughout the day. And because it's a wrap, you can even eat it on the go.

SERVES 1

1 reduced-fat pork sausage

2 reduced-fat smoked bacon medallions

1 tsp butter

2 eggs, beaten and seasoned with sea salt and freshly ground black pepper

2 tbsp baked beans

1 white tortilla wrap

Small handful of baby spinach leaves

20g reduced-fat Cheddar, grated

1. Preheat the oven to 190°C/170°C Fan/Gas 5.
2. Place the sausage on a baking tray and bake in the oven for 20–25 minutes, until cooked through.
3. Meanwhile, turn the grill to high, place the bacon on a baking tray and grill for around 7 minutes, until crisp and cooked through.
4. While the bacon is grilling, heat the butter over a medium heat in a small non-stick frying pan and, once melted, pour in the beaten eggs. Cook for around 2 minutes, stirring frequently, until lightly scrambled. Push the eggs to one side of the pan and add the beans to the other side, stirring, until heated through.
5. Open the tortilla wrap out on a plate and lay the bacon slices in the middle, so they are slightly overlapping. Lay the spinach leaves on top to cover the bacon, then slice your sausage in half lengthways and add on top.
6. Spoon over the eggs, top with the beans, then sprinkle over the cheese, so the cheese melts slightly. Wrap and enjoy!

Happier, Healthier, Tastier!

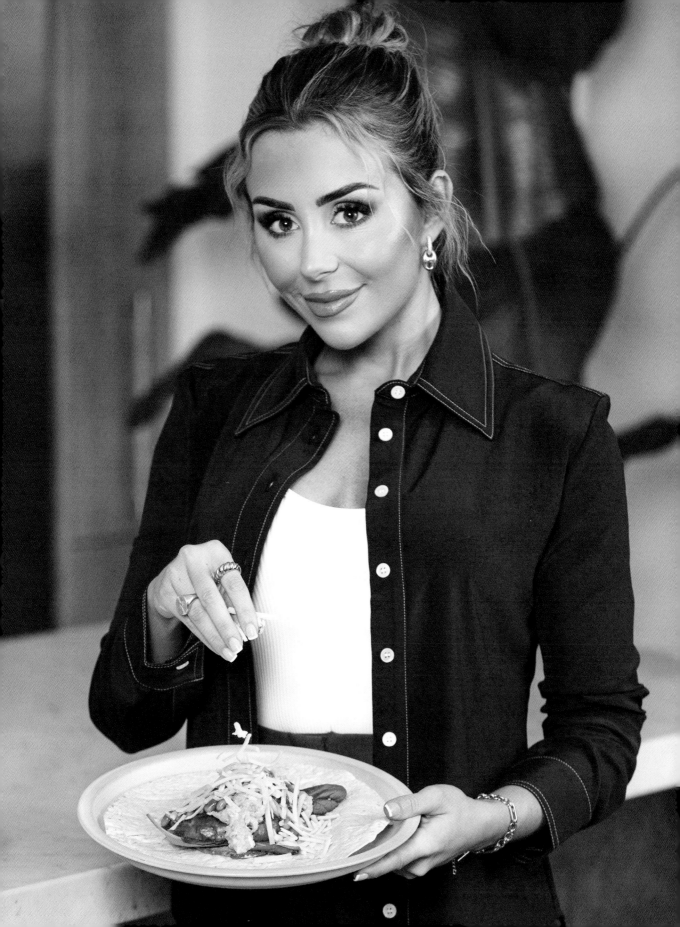

15 Minutes & Under

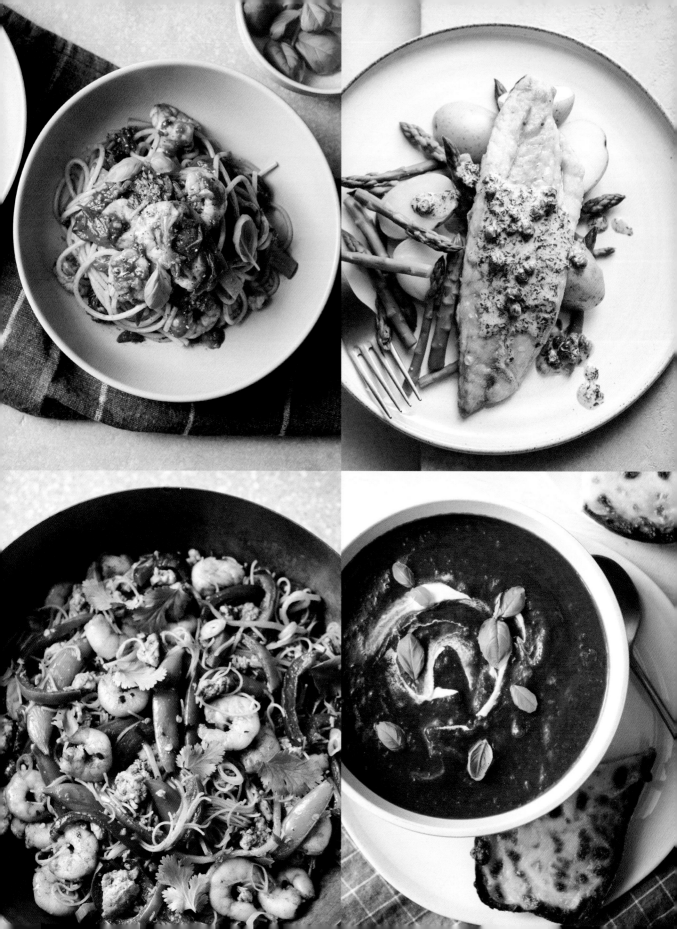

Spicy Crab Tacos
Harissa Prawn Spaghetti
Pan-fried Sea Bass with Herb Sauce
Ten-minute Creamy Tomato Soup
with Cheesy Garlic Dippers
Greek Turkey Burgers
Zingy Chicken Tacos
Sticky Hoisin Pork Chops
with Asian Slaw
Singapore Noodles
Sausage Carbonara
Tuna Orzo Salad
Pizza on Toast
Leftover Chili con Carne Quesadillas
Ham and Cheese French Toast
Quick Chorizo and Red Pepper Stew
Creamy Lemon Chicken Pasta
Pepperoni Pizza Toastie

Spicy Crab Tacos

It's taco night at home – there's no need to order a takeout when you can make these delicious, fresh ones so quickly yourself. No worries if you don't have any fresh white crab meat – just use frozen or tinned instead; the tacos will taste just as good. The pickled red onion will keep in the fridge for around two weeks once made.

Per serving:

Carbs: 13.8g

Calories: 381

Fat: 15.1g

Protein: 15.2g

SERVES 2

FOR THE PICKLED RED ONION
1 red onion, finely sliced
2 tbsp apple cider vinegar
1 tsp salt
1 tsp brown sugar

FOR THE TACOS
4 mini tortilla wraps
100g ready-to-eat fresh white crab meat
Juice of ½ lime
1 tbsp fresh coriander, roughly chopped
1 tbsp light mayonnaise
1 tsp chilli paste
1 avocado, sliced
1 tbsp fresh dill, chopped
Sea salt
Freshly ground black pepper

1. To make the pickled red onion, place the red onion, vinegar, salt and brown sugar in a small bowl and mix well to ensure the red onion is well coated. Pour over about 100ml hot water, mix again and set aside for 20 minutes to lightly pickle and soften.
2. To make the tacos, turn the flame on your smallest hob ring (if using gas; otherwise, toast in a dry pan over a medium–high heat, until warmed through) and, using a pair of tongs, carefully lay one tortilla wrap over the flame for 10 seconds, then flip and do the same on the other side. Repeat until you've lightly charred all of the wraps.
3. Place the crab meat, lime juice and coriander in a small bowl and stir to combine. Season with sea salt and black pepper.
4. In a separate small bowl, mix the mayonnaise and chilli paste together. Spoon on to the tortilla wraps and spread around with your spoon.
5. Divide the crab mixture between the wraps, then top with the sliced avocado.
6. Drain the red onion and divide between the tacos, finishing with the fresh dill.

Happier, Healthier, Tastier!

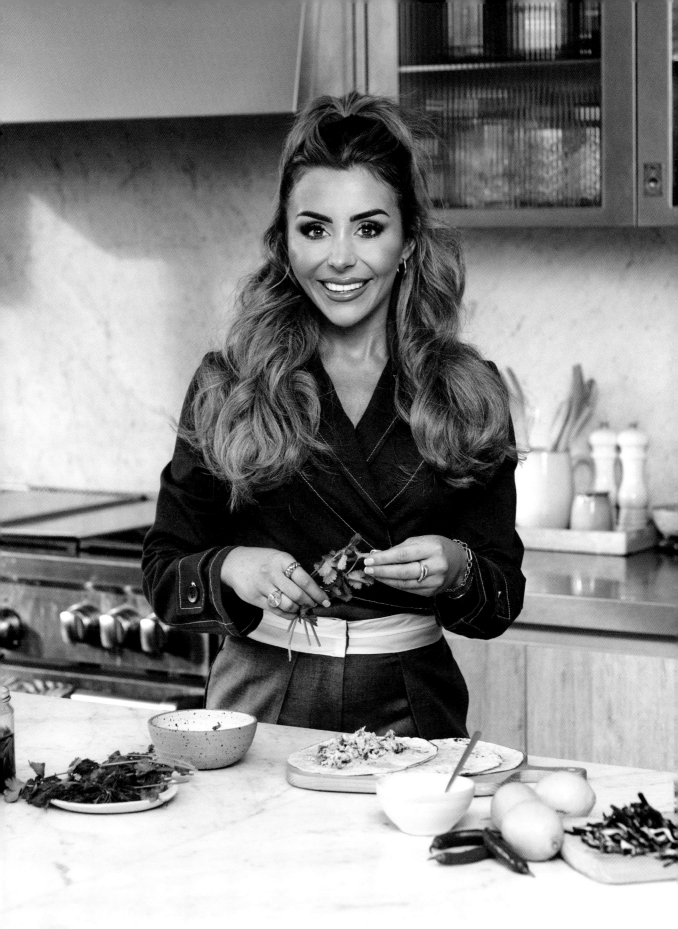

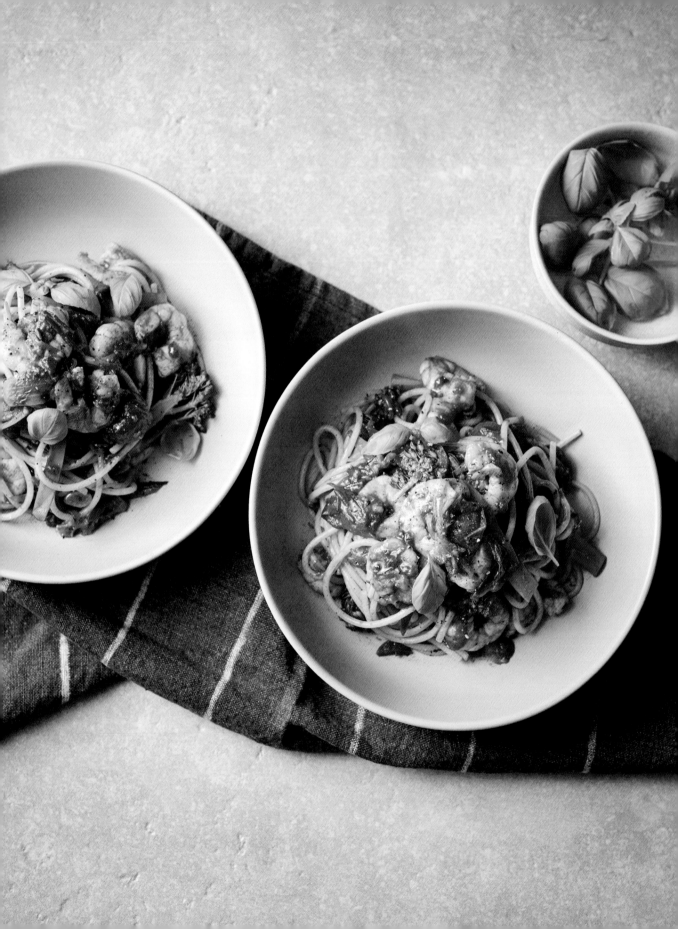

Harissa Prawn Spaghetti

Per serving:

Carbs: 70.4g

Calories: 499

Fat: 9.2g

Protein: 33.7g

This fabulous pasta dish is proof that healthy food doesn't have to be bland and boring. And it comes in at just under 500 calories per serving, so why not treat yourself. You can substitute gluten-free pasta, if desired, and it will taste – and look – just as good.

SERVES 2

150g dried spaghetti
100g Tenderstem broccoli, sliced in half
1 tbsp olive oil
1 onion, finely sliced
1 red pepper, deseeded and finely sliced
2 garlic cloves, finely sliced
100g cherry tomatoes
1 tbsp harissa paste
200g raw king prawns
½ bunch fresh basil, torn
Sea salt
Freshly ground black pepper

1. Cook the spaghetti in salted boiling water, according to the packet instructions. Add the broccoli for the final 3 minutes.
2. While your spaghetti is cooking, heat the olive oil in a large non-stick frying pan and fry the onion and red pepper for 5 minutes, until softened. Add the garlic and cherry tomatoes and fry for a further 5 minutes, squeezing the tomatoes with a wooden spoon.
3. Stir the harissa paste through the sauce and then add the prawns. The prawns are cooked as soon as they're pink (about 2 minutes). Season everything with sea salt and black pepper.
4. Drain the pasta and broccoli and stir it through the sauce. Serve with fresh basil scattered over the top.

Happier, Healthier, Tastier!

Pan-fried Sea Bass with Herb Sauce

White fish fillets are not only quick to cook but they're also high in protein and low in fat and carbs. I enjoy eating them with plain, boiled new potatoes and a low-cal creamy sauce. Delicious! You can buy fresh sea-bass fillets in many supermarkets, but if they're not available, just use sole or lemon sole instead.

Per serving:

Carbs: 28.5g

Calories: 305

Fat: 8.2g

Protein: 28g

SERVES 2

300g new potatoes, halved
125g asparagus tips
Plain flour, for dusting
2 fillets of sea bass
1 tbsp low-fat spread
1 garlic clove, crushed with the back of a knife
Juice of ½ lemon
1 tbsp reduced-fat crème fraîche
1 tbsp capers
1 tbsp finely chopped fresh parsley
1 tbsp finely chopped fresh dill
Sea salt

1. Boil the potatoes for 8–10 minutes, until cooked. Add the asparagus for the final 2 minutes of cooking. Drain and set aside.
2. While the potatoes are cooking, sprinkle a good amount of plain flour on a large plate and lightly dust the sea bass with it. Shake and tap the fish to remove most of the flour, leaving just a light dusting.
3. Heat the low-fat spread in a large non-stick frying pan over a medium heat and, once bubbling, season your fish with sea salt and place in the hot spread. Fry for 4 minutes, skin-side down, then carefully flip and fry for a further minute. Don't move the sea bass while it's in the pan (other than to flip it), as it will break up.
4. Add the garlic to the pan and, using a spoon, baste the fish with the melting garlic-infused spread.
5. Carefully remove the sea bass from the pan and keep it warm under some foil. Increase the heat under the pan and add the lemon juice, crème fraîche and a splash of water. Let it bubble for 30 seconds, then mix through the capers, parsley and dill. Serve the sauce drizzled over the sea bass, potatoes and asparagus.

Happier, Healthier, Tastier!

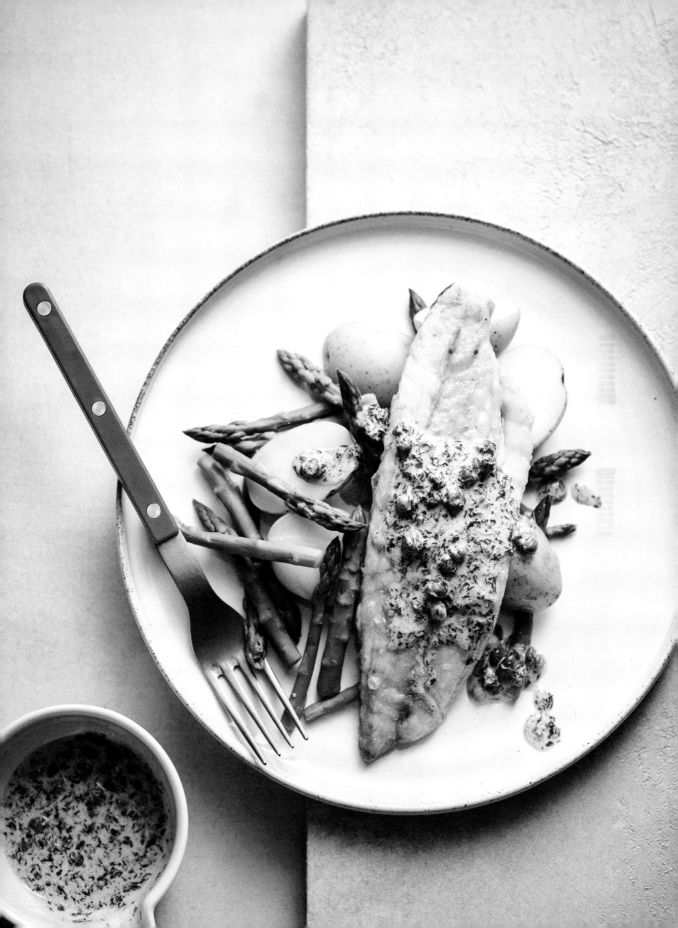

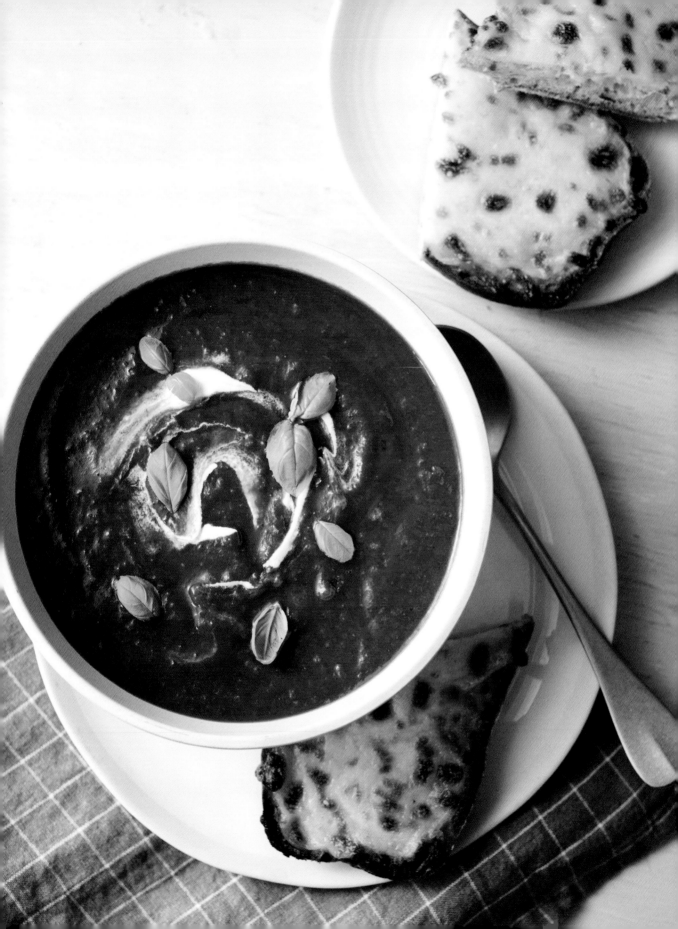

Ten-minute Creamy Tomato Soup with Cheesy Garlic Dippers ⓥ

Per serving:

Carbs: 36g

Calories: 367

Fat: 19g

Protein: 20.6g

Those packs of instant cup-a-soups in your store cupboard will become redundant when you discover this little number. It's ready in minutes and perfect for a light lunch or supper. Or you can pop the soup into a flask and the cheesy garlic dippers into a vacuum-insulated food container for a delicious, healthy packed lunch.

SERVES 2

FOR THE SOUP
1 tbsp olive oil
1 small red onion, finely sliced
2 garlic cloves, finely sliced
1 tsp dried basil
1 tsp dried oregano
1 x jar tomato passata (about 680g)
1 tbsp balsamic vinegar
½ vegetable stock pot
1 tsp honey
1 tbsp reduced-fat crème fraîche
Sea salt
Freshly ground black pepper

FOR THE CHEESY GARLIC DIPPERS
1 small ciabatta roll, sliced in half horizontally
½ garlic clove
100g reduced-fat mozzarella, grated
1 tsp balsamic vinegar
Freshly ground black pepper

1. Heat the olive oil in a large non-stick pan over a medium heat and add the red onion and garlic with the basil and oregano. Fry, stirring frequently for 2 minutes, until softened.
2. Add the passata, balsamic vinegar, stock pot, honey and a splash of hot water. Season with salt and pepper and stir well. Leave to gently bubble for 5 minutes, while you make the dippers.
3. Pop the grill on high. Place the ciabatta halves open-side up on a baking tray lined with non-stick baking paper, and rub them with the open side of the garlic. Top with the grated mozzarella and add a crack of black pepper. Grill for a couple of minutes, until golden and bubbly. Drizzle with the balsamic vinegar.
4. To finish the soup and make it extra smooth, blitz with a hand blender or leave it slightly chunky, if you prefer.
5. Remove from the heat and stir through the crème fraîche. Serve with the cheesy dippers and enjoy.

Happier, Healthier, Tastier!

Greek Turkey Burgers

Per serving:

Carbs: 34.7g

Calories: 504

Fat: 18.2g

Protein: 47.1g

Packed full of flavour and goodness, these lightly spiced burgers will bring back happy memories of warm summer days in beachside tavernas. I like to serve them in buns with a tzatziki-like mint yoghurt, salad and some salty feta and olives for a speedy supper.

SERVES 2

350g lean turkey mince
1 tbsp dried breadcrumbs
1 garlic clove, finely grated
1 tsp dried oregano
½ tsp dried chilli flakes
2 tbsp light mayonnaise
Plain flour, for dusting
   1 tbsp olive oil
1 tbsp fat-free yoghurt
1 tsp chopped fresh mint
2 burger buns
Sea salt
Freshly ground black
   pepper

TO SERVE

Lettuce leaves
Sliced red onion
Sliced tomato
50g reduced-fat feta,
   crumbled
1 tbsp black olives, halved
Slices of cucumber

1. Combine the turkey mince, dried breadcrumbs, garlic, oregano, chilli flakes, sea salt and black pepper in a bowl, along with 1 tablespoon of the mayonnaise. Mix everything with your hands for a minute, until very well combined, breaking down the meat as you go.
2. Shape the mixture into roughly 1cm-thick patties. If your patties are too sticky to handle, dust them, and your surface, with some flour.
3. Heat the olive oil in a non-stick frying pan or griddle pan over a medium–high heat and fry the patties for 4–5 minutes on each side, until cooked through.
4. While the patties are cooking, in a small bowl, combine the yoghurt, the remaining mayonnaise and the fresh mint.
5. Gently toast the insides of your burger buns and then spoon the mint yoghurt over the bottom half of each.
6. Divide the lettuce between the buns, then add a patty, some red onion and the tomato to each one. Sprinkle over the crumbled feta, black olives and cucumber slices.

Happier, Healthier, Tastier!

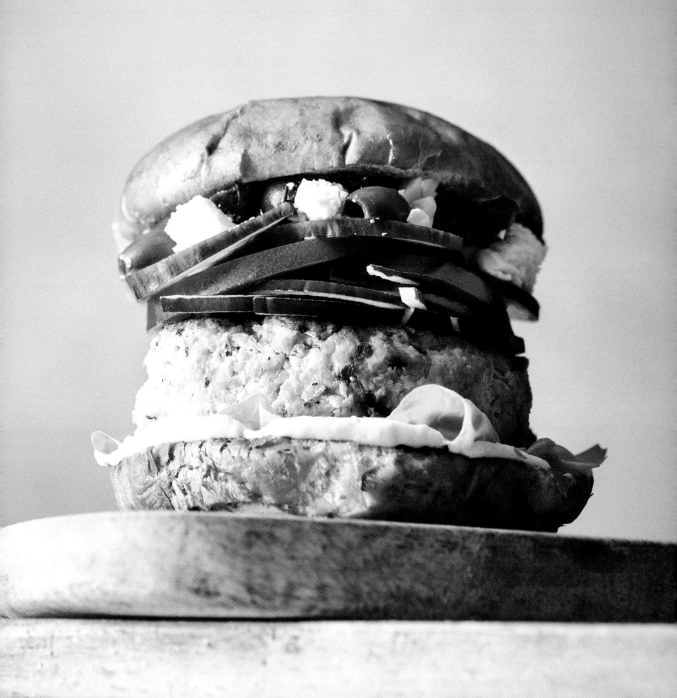

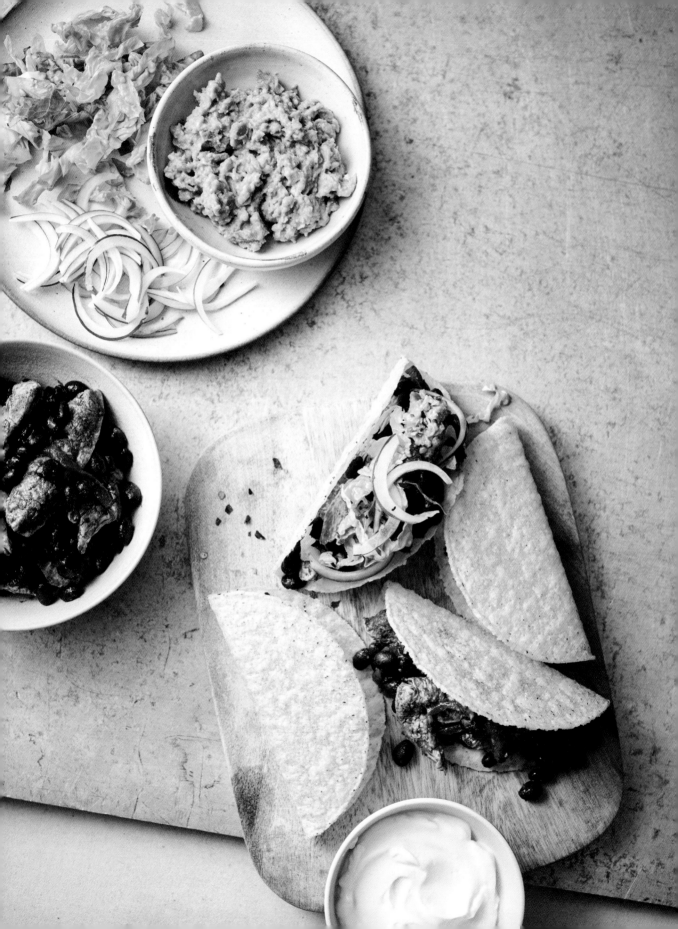

Zingy Chicken Tacos

Per serving:

Carbs: 28.1g

Calories: 388

Fat: 11.8g

Protein: 31.7g

Tonight's dinner's a wrap – and, what's more, it ticks all the boxes: it's jam packed with colour, flavour and nutritional goodness, plus everything is cooked in one pan, which saves on washing up. Your family will love these zingy tacos and they're sure to become a firm favourite on repeat.

SERVES 4

1 tbsp olive oil
400g chicken breasts, cut into strips
1 tsp smoked paprika
1 tbsp Cajun seasoning
1 × 400g tin black beans, drained
Juice of 1 lemon
1 roasted red pepper from a jar, drained and finely sliced
8 corn taco shells
1 avocado, mashed
1 red onion, finely sliced
1 Little Gem baby lettuce, finely shredded
½ tsp dried chilli flakes
4 tbsp fat-free yoghurt
Sea salt
Freshly ground black pepper

1. Heat the olive oil in a large non-stick frying pan over a medium–high heat.
2. Dust the chicken pieces in the smoked paprika and Cajun seasoning and season with sea salt and black pepper.
3. Add the chicken to the pan and fry, stirring frequently for around 6-8 minutes, until cooked through and lightly charred.
4. Add the black beans, lemon juice and sliced red pepper and give everything a toss to heat through.
5. Load the chicken mixture into the taco shells and top with the mashed avocado, onion, lettuce and chilli flakes, then top with a dollop of fat-free yoghurt.

Happier, Healthier, Tastier!

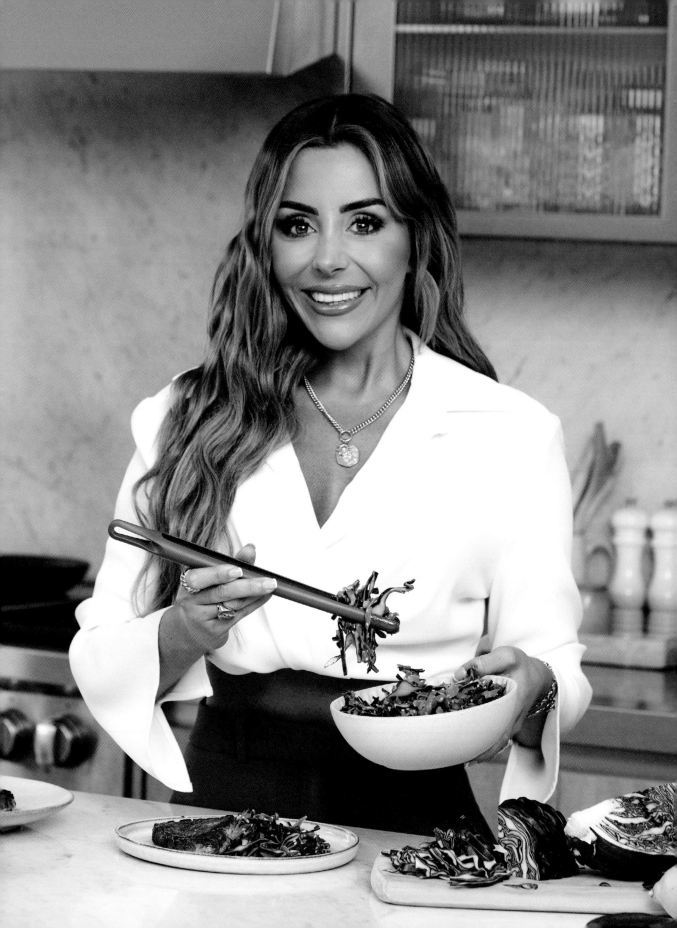

Sticky Hoisin Pork Chops with Asian Slaw

Per serving:

Carbs: 21.2g

Calories: 415

Fat: 23.9g

Protein: 28.5g

The perfect dinner if you're a fan of Chinese food! You can make the slaw in advance and rustle up the chops in less time than it takes to order a takeaway and get it delivered. Plus, it's healthier, lighter and lower in carbs and calories. We've got you covered.

SERVES 2

FOR THE HOISIN CHOPS
2 boneless pork chops
1 tsp Chinese five-spice powder
1 tsp olive oil
2 tbsp hoisin sauce

FOR THE SLAW
1 small–medium carrot, grated
1 red chilli, deseeded and finely chopped
Zest and juice of 1 lime
1cm piece of ginger, peeled and grated
¼ red cabbage, very finely sliced
1 tsp honey
1 tbsp light mayonnaise
1 tsp apple cider vinegar
1 tsp sesame seeds
1 tbsp chopped fresh coriander
2 spring onions, finely sliced

1. Take the pork chops out of the fridge 30 minutes before you want to cut them. To stop them from curling up while they're frying and to ensure even cooking, make incisions in the layer of fat at 3cm intervals.
2. Sprinkle the pork chops with the five-spice and then the rub them in the olive oil.
3. Heat a large non-stick frying pan over a medium heat, then add the pork chops to the pan, fat-side down for 3 minutes, until the fat is beginning to render and turn golden. You may need to hold the chops with a pair of tongs to stop them falling over.
4. Lay the pork chops down and fry each side for around 5 minutes, until golden brown.
5. Spoon the hoisin sauce over the chops and reduce the heat.
6. To make the slaw (this can be made ahead), simply mix all the ingredients together in a bowl.
7. Serve this dish with the pan juices drizzled over the pork chops.

Happier, Healthier, Tastier!

Singapore Noodles

Per serving:

Carbs: 50.6g

Calories: 367

Fat: 7.8g

Protein: 25.7g

Everyone will enjoy tucking into these spicy noodles. They are the perfect dish to cook when friends drop round for an informal lunch or supper. If you can't find any lean chicken mince in your local stores, just mince up some chicken-breast fillets in your food processor, chopper or blender.

SERVES 4

200g vermicelli rice noodles
1 tbsp olive oil
200g lean chicken mince
1 red pepper, deseeded and
    very finely sliced
1 green pepper, deseeded and
    very finely sliced
5 spring onions, trimmed and
    finely sliced
150g sugar snap peas
150g beansprouts
165g king prawns, cooked
1 tbsp curry powder
1 tsp ground turmeric
1 tsp dried chilli flakes
2 tbsp light soy sauce
1 tsp honey
1 bunch of fresh coriander,
    leaves torn

1. Cook the noodles according to the packet instructions.
2. Meanwhile, heat the olive oil in a large non-stick frying pan or wok over a high heat and stir-fry the chicken mince for 5 minutes, tossing frequently, until browned and nearly cooked through. Remove and set aside on a plate.
3. Add the red and green pepper, spring onions, sugar snap peas and beansprouts to the pan and stir-fry for 3–4 minutes.
4. Return the chicken mince to the pan with the prawns and sprinkle over the curry powder, ground turmeric and dried chilli flakes. Give everything a good toss to ensure it is all coated in the spices.
5. Drain the noodles and add to the pan, stirring everything through.
6. Pour the soy sauce and honey into the pan and stir well to ensure everything is coated in the delicious juice. Serve with coriander leaves on top.

Happier, Healthier, Tastier!

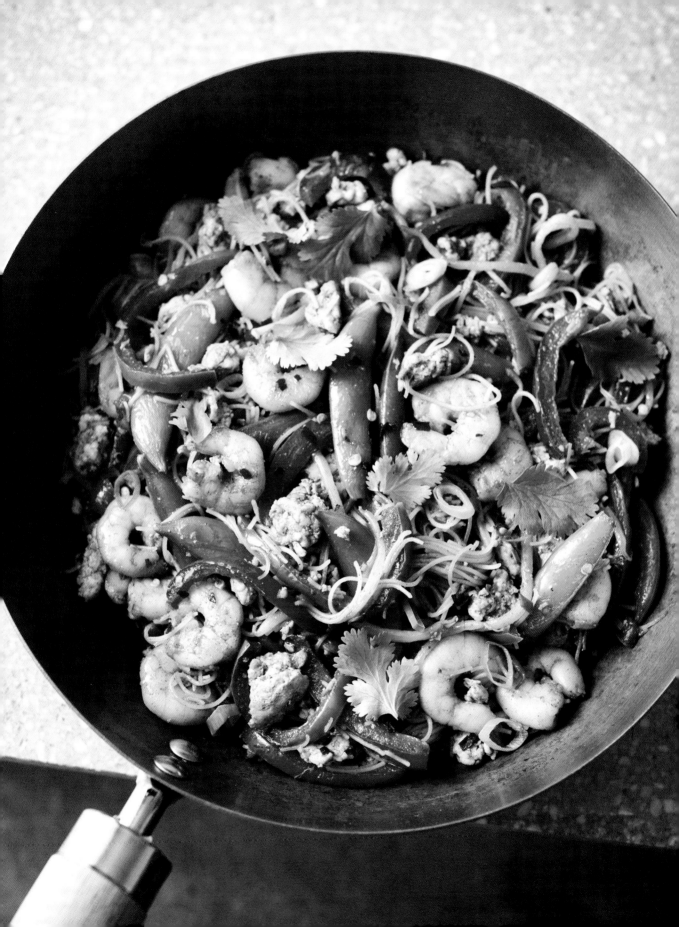

Sausage Carbonara

When it's cold outside and you want some comfort food, this is the kind of winter warmer you need. And I promise it will become a regular fixture in your life. What could be more tasty or satisfying than spaghetti carbonara with meaty sausages? And at just over 500 calories per serving, it's healthy and nutritious, too.

Per serving:

Carbs: 66.9g

Calories: 516

Fat: 11.8g

Protein: 34.1g

SERVES 2

150g spaghetti or linguine (dried)
1 tbsp olive oil
4 reduced-fat pork sausages
1 large egg
4 tbsp grated Parmesan
1 tbsp finely chopped fresh chives
Sea salt
Freshly ground black pepper

1. Cook the spaghetti in salted boiling water for 10–12 minutes, or according to the packet instructions.
2. While your spaghetti is cooking, heat the olive oil in a large non-stick frying pan over a medium heat. Squeeze the sausage meat out of the skins, then pinch small pieces of meat and gently drop them into the hot oil, browning them all over and stirring frequently.
3. Using a fork, beat the egg with 3 tablespoons of the Parmesan in a small bowl, until combined.
4. Turn the heat off under the sausages and drain the spaghetti, reserving a mug of pasta water. Add the spaghetti to the pan, along with the egg and Parmesan mixture and toss everything together.
5. Add a good splash of pasta water to the pan and continue mixing everything – the egg will cook from the heat of the pasta.
6. Serve the spaghetti with the fresh chives, the remaining Parmesan and lots of freshly cracked black pepper.

Happier, Healthier, Tastier!

Tuna Orzo Salad

Per serving:

Carbs: 44.2g

Calories: 400

Fat: 13.1g

Protein: 26.5g

Orzo pasta has become very popular, and the rice-shaped grains look great in salads. The beauty of this tasty little number is that it's so convenient, as well as easy. It uses lots of the ingredients we all keep in our store cupboards and fridges, so you don't have to do a big shop to make it.

SERVES 2

100g orzo (dry weight)
½ red onion, finely sliced
50g rocket leaves
½ x 400g tin cannellini beans, drained
1 tbsp finely chopped flat-leaf parsley
1 red chilli, deseeded and finely sliced
Juice of 1 lemon
1 tsp honey
1 tsp Dijon mustard
1 tbsp olive oil
1 × 110g tin tuna, drained
2 tbsp grated Parmesan
1 tbsp pine nuts
Sea salt
Freshly ground black pepper

1. Cook the orzo in salted boiling water for around 10 minutes, or according to the packet instructions. It's a good idea to drizzle a small amount of olive oil into the water to stop the orzo sticking together.
2. While the orzo is cooking, grab a large bowl and add the red onion, rocket, cannellini beans, parsley and red chilli. In a small jug, whisk the lemon juice, honey, Dijon mustard and olive oil together with a fork, until smooth, and season with sea salt and black pepper to taste. Flake the tuna into the bowl.
3. When the orzo is cooked, drain it in a colander and add to the salad, along with the grated Parmesan, tossing everything together. Pour over the dressing and mix well.
4. Place a small frying pan over a medium heat and lightly toast your pine nuts until golden but not dark brown (this should take 3–4 minutes), tossing frequently. Sprinkle over the salad and serve.

Happier, Healthier, Tastier!

Pizza on Toast

Per serving:

Carbs: 50.8g

Calories: 597

Fat: 20.2g

Protein: 48.6g

Yes, this sounds odd, but actually, it makes perfect sense and is such a simple way to enjoy one of your favourite foods without worrying about the calories. And it's amazingly versatile – you can add virtually any topping. Try roasted peppers, cherry tomatoes, squash, courgettes or red onion.

SERVES 1

3 slices of white baguette, sliced thickly on the diagonal (or 2 slices of ordinary white bread)

6 tbsp Italian tomato, garlic and basil passata

30g reduced-fat Cheddar, grated

40g light mozzarella, grated

5 black olives, halved

2 tbsp sweetcorn (tinned or defrosted)

80g cooked roast chicken slices

Freshly ground black pepper

1. Preheat the grill to medium–high.
2. Place the baguette (or bread) slices on a lined baking tray and lightly toast one side under the grill for a couple of minutes.
3. Remove from the grill, flip over and divide the passata between the untoasted sides. Top with the olives, sweetcorn and chicken and finally finish with the grated cheeses.
4. Grind over some black pepper and return to the grill for around 3 minutes, until the cheese is melted and the meat is lightly golden.

Happier, Healthier, Tastier!

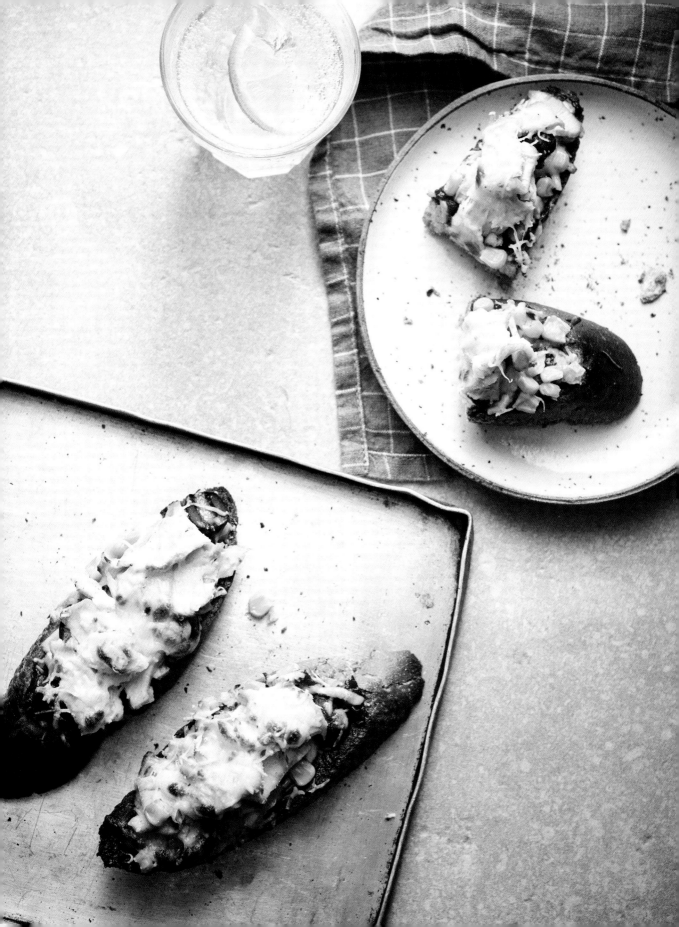

Leftover Chili con Carne Quesadillas

Per serving:

Carbs: 56.6g

Calories: 534

Fat: 17.5g

Protein: 45.4g

I hate wasting good food and am always looking for interesting ways to use and recycle leftovers. Crispy golden quesadillas are the answer to your prayers if, like me, you often have leftover chilli. This makes such a quick and easy no-fuss lunch – or you could even eat it for breakfast.

SERVES 1

1 portion leftover chili con carne (about 150g)
Low-calorie cooking spray
2 tortilla wraps
Juice of ½ lime
25g reduced-fat red Leicester, grated
1 tbsp fat-free yoghurt
1 tbsp chopped fresh coriander

1. Heat the chili in a small saucepan over a medium heat, until hot.
2. Heat a non-stick frying pan over a medium–high heat and spray with low-calorie cooking spray.
3. Place one tortilla wrap in the pan. Add the chili on top of the wrap, then squeeze over the lime juice and top with the cheese.
4. Top with the other tortilla wrap and leave the quesadilla to cook for 2–3 minutes, until the bottom is golden.
5. Carefully flip the quesadilla and cook for a further minute, until the cheese has melted.
6. Mix the yoghurt with the chopped coriander and use as a dipping sauce, to serve.

Happier, Healthier, Tastier!

Ham and Cheese French Toast

Per serving:

Carbs: 41.2g

Calories: 492

Fat: 20.5g

Protein: 32.9g

French toast is one of the ultimate comfort foods and my special variation on the classic recipe is no exception. I like to add ham and grated cheese to give it a real kick and then serve it drizzled with some hot sauce – sriracha works well.

SERVES 1

1 large egg, beaten
2 slices of thick white bread
2 thick slices of roast ham
25g reduced-fat Cheddar, grated
Low-calorie cooking spray
1 tbsp low-fat olive oil spread
Sea salt

1. Place the beaten egg in a shallow bowl, then season with some sea salt.
2. Make a sandwich as you usually would with the bread, ham and cheese. Sit the sandwich in the egg and let it soak for 20 seconds, then flip and do the same again on the other side.
3. Spray a non-stick frying pan with low-calorie cooking spray and heat the olive spread over a medium heat. Add the sandwich to the pan and fry for 3 minutes, until it is golden on the bottom, then flip over and fry for a further 2–3 minutes.
4. Serve with your favourite sauce.

Happier, Healthier, Tastier!

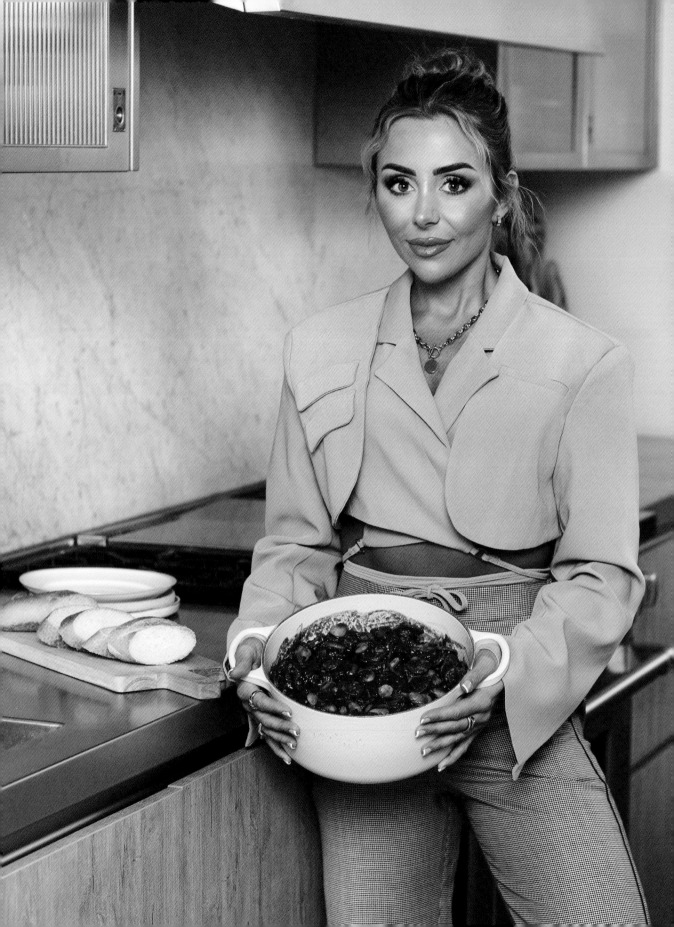

Quick Chorizo and Red Pepper Stew

Per serving:

Carbs: 24.2g

Calories: 350

Fat: 17.2g

Protein: 21.3g

Why not cook up a storm today with this Spanish-style stew? It's so delicious and tastes even better the next day, so I like to keep a couple of portions in an airtight container in the fridge or freezer for an easy supper when I'm in a hurry or don't feel like cooking. It's perfect served with fresh crusty baguette for a fuller meal, too. Get your ingredients ready before you begin preparing this to make it extra speedy!

SERVES 4

1 tsp olive oil
1 reduced-fat chorizo ring, finely sliced
1 red onion, finely sliced
2 garlic cloves, finely chopped
1 × 480g jar roasted red peppers, drained and rinsed
1 heaped tsp smoked paprika
1 × 400g tin chopped tomatoes
1 × 400g tin butter beans, drained
150ml hot chicken stock
1 tsp honey
Sea salt
Freshly ground black pepper

1. Heat the olive oil in a deep saucepan over a medium–high heat and add the chorizo and red onion with a sprinkling of sea salt and black pepper. Fry for 3–4 minutes, until the onion has softened and the chorizo has begun releasing its delicious golden oil.
2. Add the garlic and red peppers and stir everything well. Fry for a further 2 minutes.
3. Sprinkle in the smoked paprika and stir well for 1 minute.
4. Add the chopped tomatoes, butter beans, stock and honey and increase the heat.
5. Once boiling, reduce the heat to medium and leave to bubble for around 8 minutes, until thickened and delicious!

Happier, Healthier, Tastier!

Creamy Lemon Chicken Pasta

Per serving:

Carbs: 59g

Calories: 458

Fat: 9.8g

Protein: 28g

If you're stuck for ideas for tonight's supper, then look no further. I love to make this wonderfully soothing, low-cal pasta when I'm feeling tired at the end of a long and busy day. It's so delish and helps me to wind down and really relax.

SERVES 4

300g dried tagliatelle (or your choice of pasta)

2 boneless, skinless chicken breasts

3 tbsp plain flour

1 tbsp olive oil

Juice of 1 lemon, plus an extra squeeze to serve

2 tbsp reduced-fat crème fraîche

40g Parmesan, grated

Sea salt

Freshly ground black pepper

1. Cook the pasta in salted, boiling water, according to the packet instructions.
2. Meanwhile, place your hand on top of a chicken breast and carefully slice through it horizontally. Repeat with the second breast, so you're left with 4 thinner cutlets of chicken.
3. Sprinkle the flour out on to a plate, then lightly dredge the chicken cutlets in the flour and shake off any excess.
4. Heat the olive oil in a non-stick frying pan over a medium–high heat and fry the chicken breasts for 2–3 minutes on each side, until cooked through, ensuring no pink remains and the juices run clear. Remove from the heat and squeeze over the juice of half the lemon. Set aside to rest.
5. Drain the pasta, reserving a small amount of the cooking water, then return to the pan, along with the rest of the lemon juice, crème fraîche, Parmesan and a splash of the pasta water. Season well with black pepper and toss everything together, so the pasta is well coated.
6. Serve the pasta with a chicken cutlet on top and an extra squeeze of lemon juice.

Happier, Healthier, Tastier!

Pepperoni Pizza Toastie

Another super-speedy pizza for when you're in a hurry. And you don't have to do a big shop because you'll have most of the ingredients in your store cupboard and fridge.

Per serving:
Carbs: 19.9g
Calories: 553
Fat: 16.7g
Protein: 17.2g

SERVES 2
50g reduced-fat Cheddar, grated
50g reduced-fat grated mozzarella
2 tbsp low-fat spread
4 slices of white bread
2 tbsp tomato passata with herbs
8 slices of reduced-fat pepperoni or salami
½ bunch of basil leaves
Freshly ground black pepper

1. Combine the Cheddar and mozzarella in a small bowl and season with black pepper.
2. Spread half the low-fat spread over two slices of bread on one side. Lay these two slices on a plate with the buttered side down.
3. Spread the tomato passata over the top of the two pieces of bread, then add two slices of pepperoni to each. Sprinkle the cheese mixture over the pepperoni, then add the remaining pepperoni and the basil leaves. Top with the remaining slices of bread.
4. Heat the remaining low-fat spread in a non-stick frying pan over a medium heat and fry the sandwiches for 2–3 minutes on each side, until the toast is golden and the cheese has melted.
5. To make this easier, you can use a weight, such as another pan or something heavy, to push the sandwiches down – this will help them to cook more evenly.

Happier, Healthier, Tastier!

Fakeaways

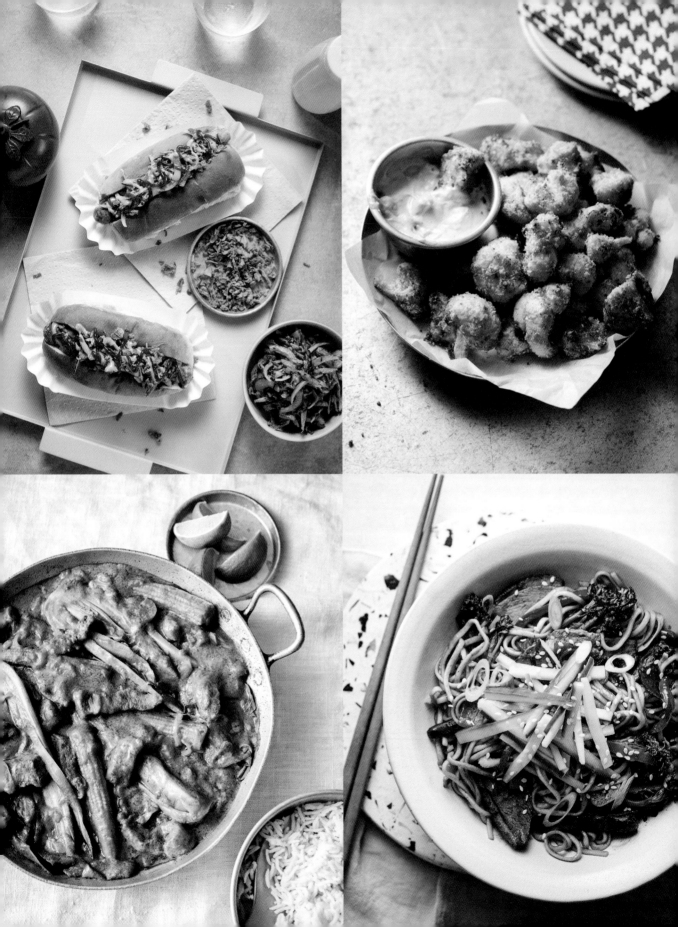

Crispy Duck Stir-fry
Guilt-free Prawn Toast
Sticky Asian Glazed Meatballs
Sriracha Popcorn Cauliflower
Beef Panang Curry
Peri-peri Chicken Wrap
Thai Chicken Burger
Sunrise Burger
Beef Yakitori Skewers
Pulled Pork Nachos
Fish-fillet Burger
Crispy Pork Souvlaki
Grilled Salmon-loaded Gyros
Chinese Char Siu Pork
with Special Fried Rice
Loaded Hot Dogs
Melt-in-the-middle Fishcakes
Crispy Halloumi Fajitas
Creamy Prawn Laksa
Cheese and Onion Pasties
Tandoori Salmon Burger

Crispy Duck Stir-fry

Per serving:

Carbs: 65.1g

Calories: 600

Fat: 23.5g

Protein: 29.5g

Crispy duck is always one of the most popular choices on the menu in any Chinese restaurant . . . but, unfortunately, it's usually loaded with fat and unwanted calories. My version tastes better than any takeaway and it's much healthier, too, with lots of yummy vegetables.

SERVES 2

1 tsp Chinese five-spice powder
2 duck breasts, skin scored with a sharp knife in a criss-cross pattern
1 tsp vegetable oil
2 nests of egg noodles
1 red onion, roughly chopped
1 red pepper, deseeded and finely sliced
100g Tenderstem broccoli
2 garlic cloves, finely grated
1 red chilli, deseeded and finely sliced
2 tbsp hoisin sauce, mixed with 1 tbsp water
4 spring onions, trimmed and finely sliced
½ cucumber, halved lengthways, deseeded, then sliced into matchsticks
1 tbsp sesame seeds (optional)
Sea salt
Freshly ground black pepper

1. Preheat the oven to 200°C/ 180°C Fan/Gas 6.
2. Sprinkle the five-spice powder over the duck breasts and season with salt and pepper.
3. Heat the oil in a large non-stick frying pan or wok over a high heat and, once smoking, add the duck breasts skin-side down. Allow to fry for 4–5 minutes until the skin is brown and crisp, then flip and fry on the other side for a further minute.
4. Transfer the duck breasts to a lined baking tray, skin-side up, and cook in the oven for 5 minutes until they're cooked through – pink is good!
5. While the duck breasts are roasting, cook the egg noodles in boiling water, according to the packet instructions.
6. Turn the heat to high under the pan you used for the duck (there should be residual oil in the pan). Stir-fry the red onion and red pepper until softened and lightly golden.
7. Add the Tenderstem broccoli and fry for a further 2–3 minutes, stirring frequently.
8. When the duck breasts are cooked, slice and add to the pan, along with the garlic and chilli, tossing everything together.
9. Pour in the hoisin sauce and water and add the spring onions. Toss everything to coat. Add the noodles and toss them through.
10. Serve with the cucumber on top and the sesame seeds sprinkled over (if using).

Happier, Healthier, Tastier!

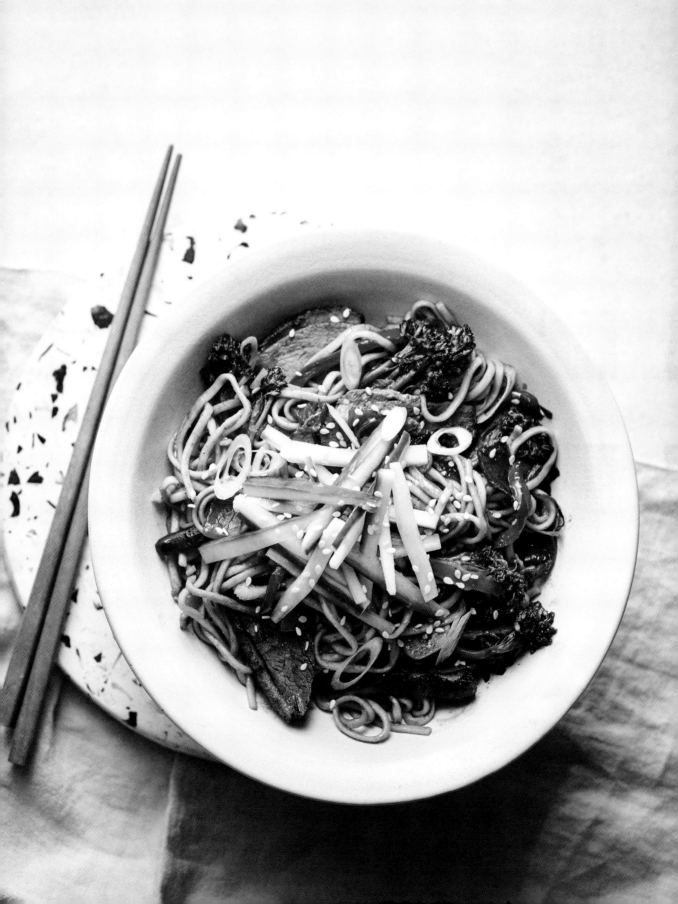

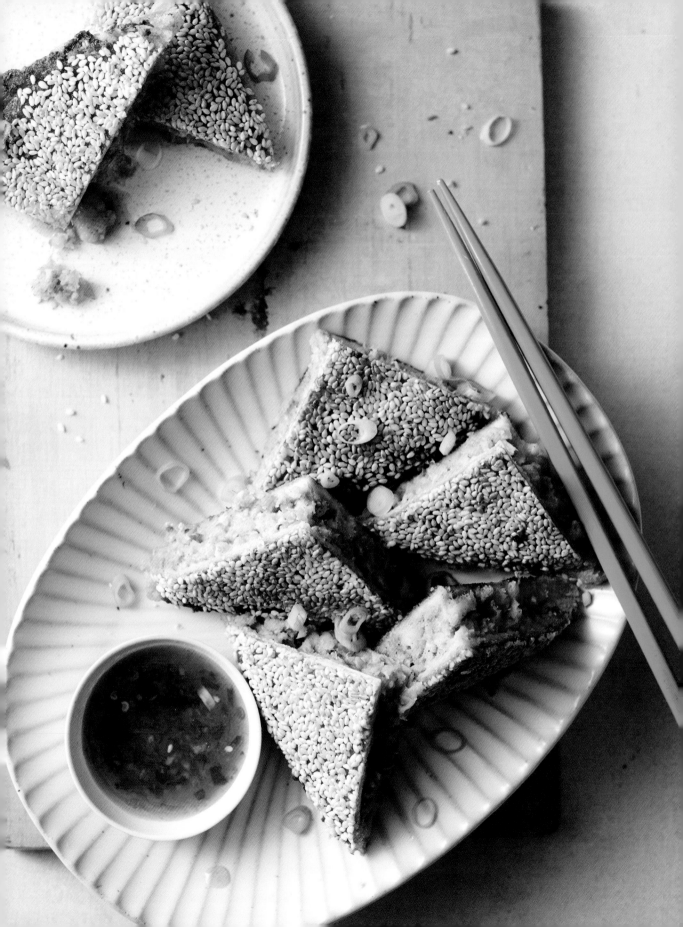

Guilt-free Prawn Toast

Per serving:

Carbs: 21.6g

Calories: 279

Fat: 12.3g

Protein: 19.6g

Prawn toast is always so delicious to order in, but the chances are it's been deep-fried and loaded with fat and carbs. Luckily, I've come up with a guilt-free alternative, which is healthier and just as tasty, so you can continue to enjoy one of your favourite treats.

SERVES 2

165g raw king prawns

4 spring onions, 2 roughly chopped and 2 finely sliced

1 garlic clove

2 tsp minced ginger

1 tsp cornflour

1 egg, separated

½ tsp Chinese five-spice powder

1 tsp soy sauce

4 slices of white bread, crusts removed

3 tbsp sesame seeds

Low-calorie cooking spray

Chilli jam or sweet chilli sauce, to serve

1. Place the prawns, the chopped spring onions, garlic and ginger in a blender. Blitz, until finely minced – you don't want a purée.
2. Transfer to a large bowl and stir in the cornflour, egg yolk, five-spice powder and soy sauce, until well combined.
3. Spread the prawn mixture over two slices of bread, then place the other slices on top. Brush all sides of the sandwich with the egg white, then sprinkle the sesame seeds over the top, pressing them in, so they don't fall off when you're frying the sandwiches.
4. Heat the low-calorie cooking spray in a non-stick frying pan over a medium heat and fry the sandwiches for 2–3 minutes on each side, until cooked through. It helps to pop something slightly heavy on top of the sandwich to weigh it down, so it cooks more evenly.
5. Sprinkle the sliced spring onions over the top and serve with chilli jam or sweet chilli sauce.

Happier, Healthier, Tastier!

Sticky Asian Glazed Meatballs

Per serving:

Carbs: 27.5g

Calories: 340

Fat: 10.9g

Protein: 33.3g

Can you believe it? These delish meatballs are not only a really healthy low-calorie supper, but they are ready in, literally, minutes! Less time than it takes to order and deliver a takeaway from your local restaurant. And you can ring the changes by substituting minced chicken, turkey or beef for the pork.

SERVES 4

300g basmati rice
500g lean pork mince
2 garlic cloves, finely grated
3 tbsp finely chopped fresh
   coriander
Thumb-sized piece of ginger,
   finely grated
2 limes – zest and juice of 1,
   plus wedges to serve
2 tsp soy sauce
1 tsp fish sauce
2 tbsp honey
1 tbsp olive oil

TO SERVE

Spring onions, finely sliced
Little Gem lettuce leaves
Sesame seeds, for sprinkling

1. Cook the rice according to the packet instructions.
2. To make the meatballs, grab a large bowl and combine the pork mince, garlic, coriander, ginger, lime juice, 1 teaspoon of the soy sauce and the fish sauce. Roll the mixture into balls of your desired size – it should make 20–25.
3. In a small bowl, whisk together the remaining soy sauce, lime zest and honey: this is your glaze.
4. Heat the olive oil in a large non-stick frying pan over a medium heat and, once hot, add the meatballs. To get them browned and cooked through, you'll need to fry them for 8–10 minutes. Don't let the heat become too high, otherwise the outsides will burn. The larger they are, the longer they will take to cook.
5. When the meatballs are cooked through, add the glaze to the pan and stir to ensure the balls are all evenly coated.
6. Pile the rice into bowls and spoon over the delicious sticky meatballs. Serve with lime wedges, the spring onions, lettuce leaves and sesame seeds sprinkled over.

Happier, Healthier, Tastier!

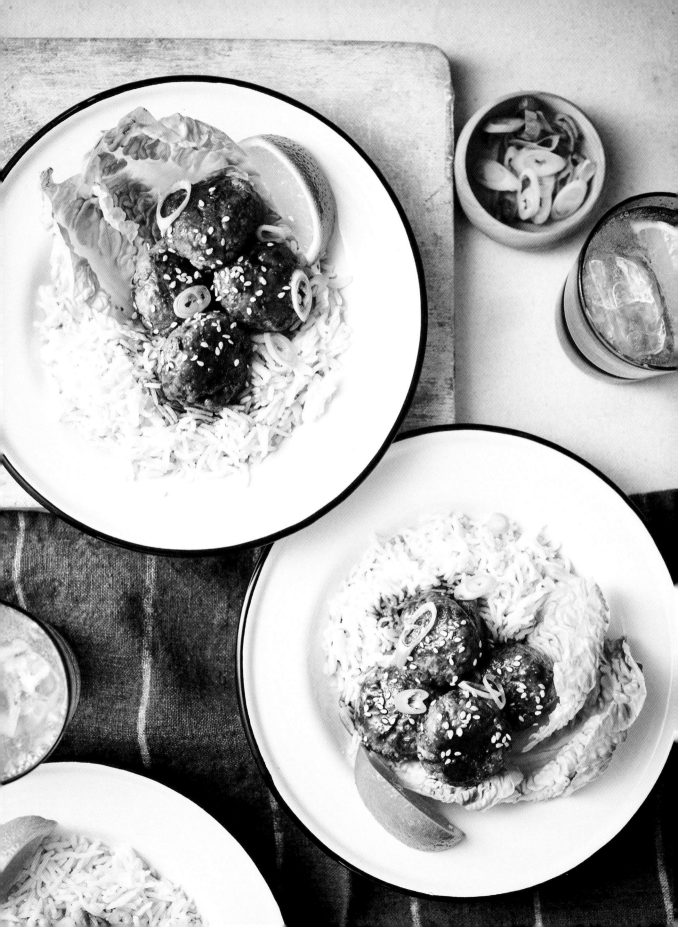

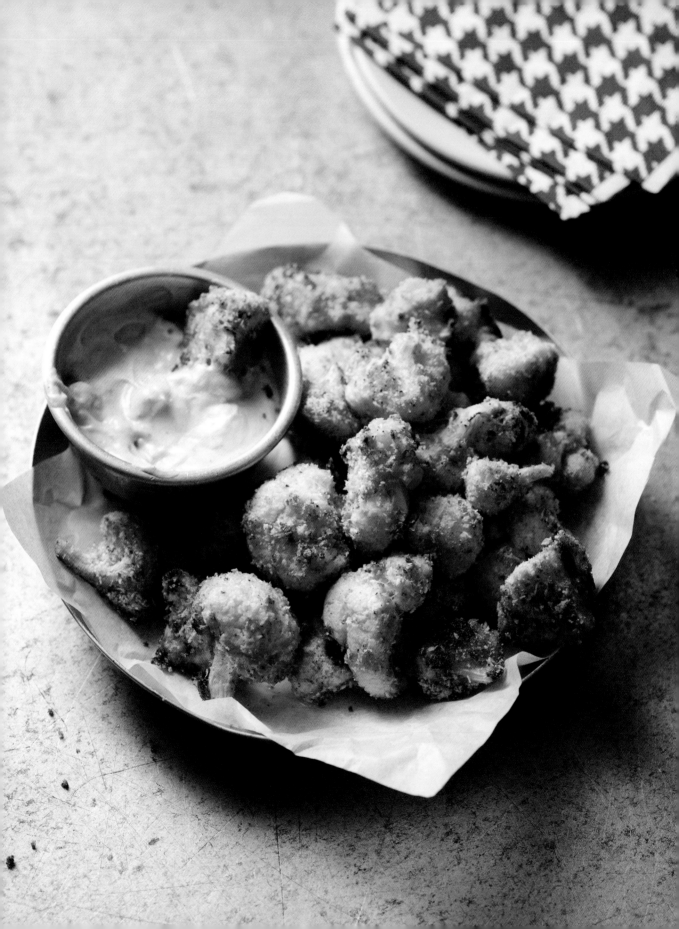

Sriracha Popcorn Cauliflower Ⓥ

Per serving:

Carbs: 22.5g

Calories: 189

Fat: 7.3g

Protein: 8.7g

Here's my low-cal take on popcorn cauliflower, so you can enjoy it at home as a healthy snack, eat it as a side or serve it to your guests with pre-dinner drinks. And the sriracha yoghurt and mayo dip adds a fabulous finishing touch. Super simple and delicious.

SERVES 4 (OR 2 HUNGRY SNACKERS!)

1 cauliflower, sliced into small florets
70g panko breadcrumbs
50g reduced-fat Parmesan, grated
1 tsp smoked paprika
1 tsp garlic powder
1 tsp onion powder
1 egg, beaten
Low-calorie cooking spray
4 tbsp light mayonnaise
1 tbsp fat-free yoghurt
½ garlic clove, finely grated
2 tsp sriracha sauce
Sea salt
Freshly ground black pepper

1. Preheat the oven to 210°C/190°C Fan/Gas 6–7.
2. Cook the cauliflower for 4 minutes in a saucepan of boiling water over a high heat, then drain and leave to cool.
3. In a large bowl, mix the breadcrumbs, Parmesan, smoked paprika and garlic and onion powders. Season well with sea salt and black pepper.
4. In a separate large bowl, mix the drained cauliflower with the egg. Sprinkle in the breadcrumb mixture and toss to evenly coat the cauliflower.
5. Transfer the coated cauliflower to a baking tray and spray well with low-calorie cooking spray.
6. Bake for 25–30 minutes, until golden and cooked through.
7. Meanwhile, grab a small bowl and whisk together the mayonnaise, yoghurt, garlic and sriracha sauce, until combined. Use this as your dipping sauce.

Happier, Healthier, Tastier!

Beef Panang Curry

Friday night is curry night – so instead of ordering a takeaway from the local Indian, try cooking this little gem at home. You'll have a delicious creamy curry in under thirty minutes. To make it more substantial, serve it with plain, boiled basmati rice, which will add 130 calories and 27g carbs per 100g portion.

Per serving:

Carbs: 10.5g	
Calories: 396	
Fat: 22.5g	
Protein: 34.1g	

SERVES 4

1 tbsp olive oil
500g lean diced beef
1 tbsp plain flour
2 small onions, finely sliced
4 tbsp Panang curry paste
1 × 400g tin light coconut milk
4 tbsp crunchy peanut butter
1 tsp fish sauce
1 × 400g tin chopped tomatoes
200g pak choi, halved lengthways
150g baby corn
Juice of 1 lime
Sea salt
Freshly ground black pepper

1. Heat the olive oil in a large non-stick frying pan over a high heat and dust the beef in the flour. Season with sea salt and black pepper.
2. Add the beef to the pan and brown on all sides, then remove with a slotted spoon and set aside.
3. Add the onions to the pan and fry for 4–5 minutes over a medium heat, until softened and lightly golden.
4. Stir in the curry paste for 1 minute, then add the beef back to the frying pan.
5. Pour in the coconut milk, peanut butter, fish sauce and chopped tomatoes and bring to the boil. Reduce the heat immediately to a simmer and leave to bubble for 10–15 minutes.
6. Add the pak choi and baby corn and cook for a further 5 minutes.
7. Serve with a squeeze of lime juice over the top.

Happier, Healthier, Tastier!

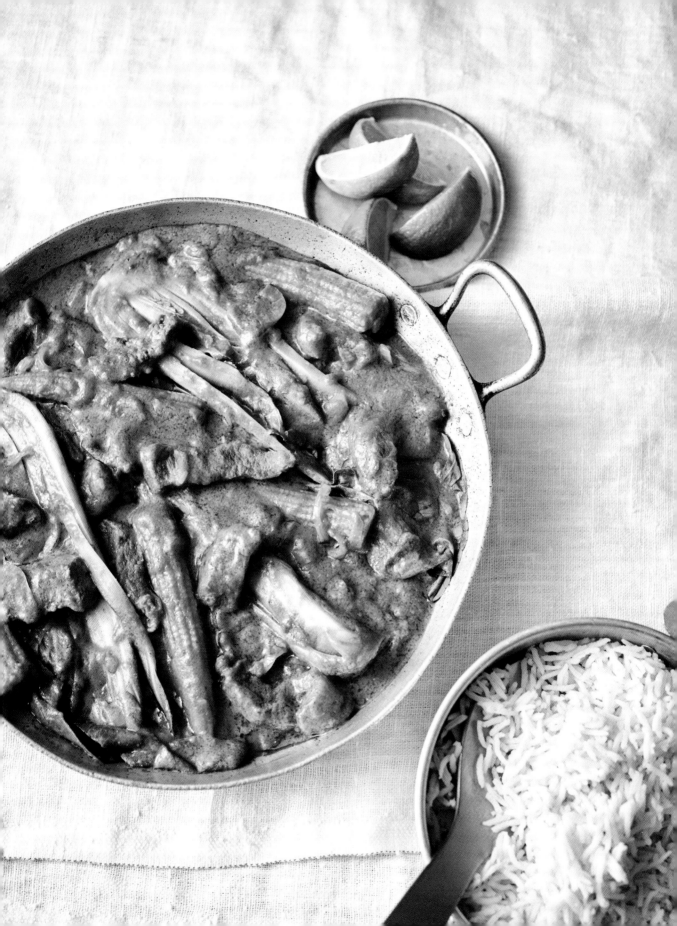

Peri-peri Chicken Wrap

Meals don't come easier than this! Just pop everything in a pan with a dash of spicy peri-peri seasoning, wrap it up with some healthy salad and, hey presto – dinner is served. No need to order a takeaway when you can make these so quickly and easily.

Per serving:

Carbs: 25.4g

Calories: 407

Fat: 10.1g

Protein: 42.3g

MAKES 2

Low-calorie cooking spray
1 red onion, finely sliced
1 red pepper, deseeded and finely sliced
250g chicken breast mini fillets
1 tbsp peri-peri seasoning
1 tsp smoked paprika
1 tsp ground cumin
1 tbsp lazy garlic (paste from a jar)
3 tbsp light mayonnaise
2 tortilla wraps
2 tbsp chilli jam
Juice of ½ lemon
Spinach leaves, to serve
Iceberg lettuce leaves, to serve
¼ cucumber, sliced

1. Spray a non-stick frying pan with the cooking spray over a medium heat and add the red onion, red pepper and chicken breast fillets. Sprinkle over the peri-peri seasoning, smoked paprika and cumin and fry the chicken and vegetables for around 5–8 minutes, until the chicken is cooked through and the vegetables are tender. Add the garlic and stir, frying for 1 minute.
2. Spread the mayonnaise over the wraps and then spoon over the chilli jam.
3. When the chicken is cooked, squeeze over the lemon juice and give everything a good stir.
4. Add the spinach and lettuce leaves to the wrap, then arrange the cucumber slices over the top.
5. Load the wraps with the spicy chicken, onion and pepper, then roll them up and enjoy!

Happier, Healthier, Tastier!

Thai Chicken Burger

My all-time favourite burger! I adore Thai food and love experimenting with their classic spices, herbs and sauces. Here, they've all come together to make super-delish burgers that you're gonna love. I guarantee they'll become a permanent feature in your repertoire.

MAKES 4
400g chicken mince
2 tbsp dried breadcrumbs
1 garlic clove, finely grated
Thumb-sized piece of ginger, peeled and finely grated
1 tsp fresh lime zest
½ bunch fresh coriander, finely chopped
1 egg, beaten
1 tbsp olive oil
4 brioche burger buns, halved
4 tbsp fat-free yoghurt
Juice of ½ lime
½ cucumber, cut into ribbons using a speed peeler
1 carrot, cut into ribbons using a speed peeler
4 tbsp sweet chilli sauce
Sea salt
Freshly ground black pepper

1. Grab a large bowl and combine the chicken mince, breadcrumbs, garlic, ginger, lime zest, coriander and egg. Season well with sea salt and black pepper. It is best to work this mixture with your hands for a couple of minutes, as this will help to ensure the patties don't fall apart when you fry them.
2. Shape the mixture into 4 burger patties, as neatly as possible.
3. Heat the olive oil in a large non-stick frying pan over a medium heat and fry the patties for around 5 minutes on each side, until cooked through. Make sure they're piping hot in the middle.
4. Lightly toast your brioche buns, then mix the yoghurt and lime juice together and spoon over the bases of the buns.
5. Add a chicken burger to each bun and top with the cucumber and carrot ribbons.
6. Add a dollop of sweet chilli sauce to the top of each one, finish with the bun halves and enjoy!

Happier, Healthier, Tastier!

Sunrise Burger

Per serving:

Carbs: 46g

Calories: 598

Fat: 19.8g

Protein: 53.8g

Most of us never tire of burgers, and who would have thought that there are so many delicious ways of flavouring them. To make these colourful ones, I've layered up chicken thighs with peri-peri mayo, chilli jam and cheese. They're sunrise on a plate!

MAKES 2
Low-calorie cooking spray
1 tbsp plain flour
4 boneless, skinless chicken thighs
4 tbsp light mayonnaise
2 tbsp peri-peri sauce
2 soft burger buns
1 Little Gem lettuce, leaves trimmed
2 tbsp chilli jam
2 reduced-fat cheese singles
Sea salt
Freshly ground black pepper

1. Preheat the oven to 200°C/180°C Fan/Gas 6.
2. Spray a large non-stick frying pan with cooking spray over a medium–high heat.
3. Put the plain flour on a plate and fork through some sea salt and black pepper. Lightly dust the chicken thighs with the flour.
4. Fry the chicken thighs for 3 minutes on each side, until lightly crisp, then transfer to a baking tray and bake in the oven for 8–10 minutes, until cooked through – when no pink remains and the juices run clear.
5. While your chicken thighs are roasting, mix the mayonnaise with the peri-peri sauce and set aside.
6. Halve and lightly toast your burger buns, then add a layer of the mayonnaise to the base of each bun. Top with the lettuce leaves.
7. Remove the chicken from the oven and place two thighs on each bun base, one on top of the other.
8. Spoon over any remaining mayonnaise, then the chilli jam and top off with a cheese single and the tops of the buns.

Happier, Healthier, Tastier!

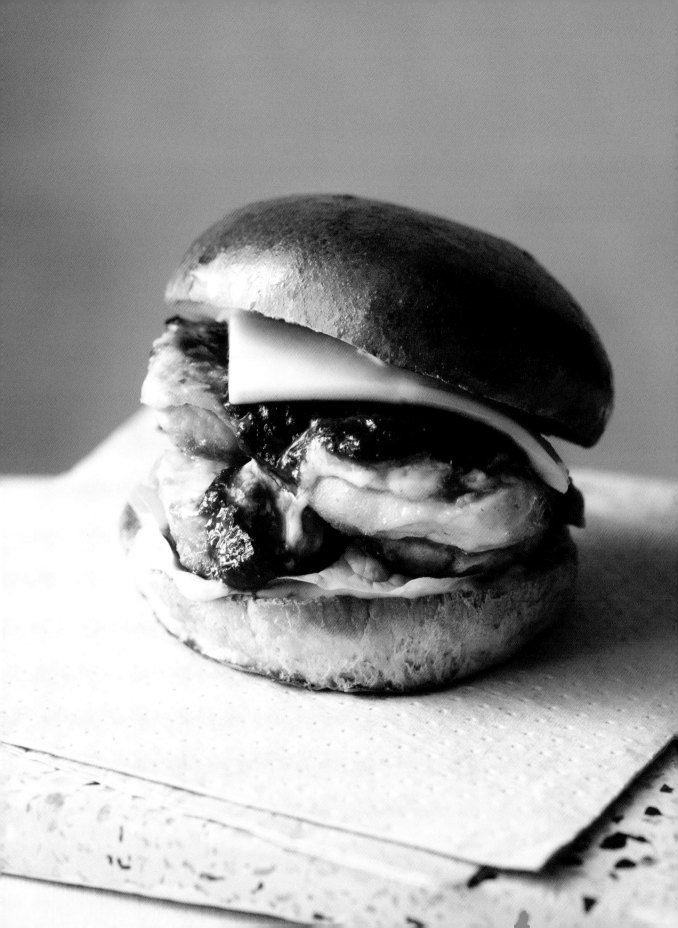

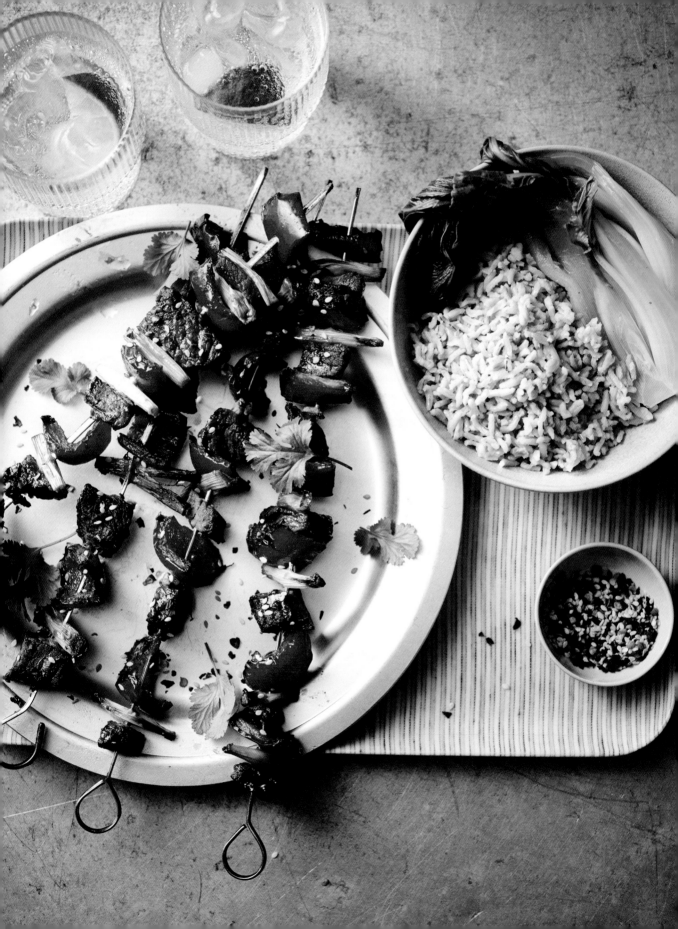

Beef Yakitori Skewers

I haven't forgotten all you Japanese food lovers – I'm a fan, too! These tasty beef kebabs are served with crunchy, nutty-flavoured brown rice, which is healthier and higher in fibre than white rice. If you use wooden or bamboo skewers instead of metal ones, remember to soak them in warm water for at least ten minutes before threading with the beef and vegetables. This will stop them burning under the hot grill.

Per serving:

Carbs: 43.9g

Calories: 341

Fat: 6.5g

Protein: 25.8g

SERVES 4

300g brown rice
350g diced beef
8 spring onions, sliced to a similar thickness to your beef
2 red peppers, deseeded and cut into chunks – again, similar size to your beef
150g sticky yakitori sauce
2 pak choi, halved lengthways
½ bunch fresh coriander, torn
1 tsp chilli flakes, to serve
2 tbsp sesame seeds, for sprinkling

1. Cook the brown rice according to the packet instructions, then drain and set aside.
2. Meanwhile, in a large bowl, mix the beef, spring onions, red peppers and yakitori sauce, ensuring everything is coated.
3. Preheat the grill to high.
4. Grab some metal skewers and assemble them by first adding a piece of beef, then spring onion and then red pepper. Keep going until you've used up all the ingredients – it should make around 8 skewers.
5. Transfer the skewers to a foil-lined baking tray and grill for around 3 minutes on each side. Keep brushing the leftover sauce over them as they grill.
6. Boil the pak choi in boiling water for 3–4 minutes, until tender but still slightly crunchy.
7. Serve the delicious skewers on the rice with the pak choi, and top with the fresh coriander, chilli flakes and sesame seeds.

Happier, Healthier, Tastier!

Pulled Pork Nachos

Per serving:

Carbs: 37.4g

Calories: 595

Fat: 26.8g

Protein: 32.4g

Yes, it's a long list of ingredients, but you should have all the spices and sauces in your store cupboard (see page 10), so don't let that put you off making these scrummy nachos. Perfect for a cosy family supper or for sharing with friends.

SERVES 5

1 tsp olive oil
1 red onion, finely sliced
2 garlic cloves, grated
1 tsp hot chilli powder
1 tsp ground cumin
1 tsp ground cinnamon
1 tsp cayenne pepper
1 tsp smoked paprika
60g tomato ketchup
2 tbsp BBQ sauce
1 tbsp treacle
60ml white wine (or apple cider) vinegar
300ml chicken stock
500g pork tenderloin, cut into 4 equal pieces
200g salted tortilla chips
50g reduced-fat Cheddar, grated
50g reduced-fat mozzarella, grated
½ bunch of fresh coriander, leaves torn
150g tinned sweetcorn, drained
1 avocado, sliced
1 lime, cut into wedges

1. Heat the oil in a large non-stick frying pan and fry the red onion for 5 minutes, until softened and lightly golden. Add the garlic and fry for a further 2 minutes.
2. Add the spices, stir well and cook them out for 1 minute.
3. Add the ketchup, BBQ sauce, treacle, vinegar and stock and stir well.
4. Carefully add the pork, cover and simmer over a low heat for around 25 minutes, until the pork is just cooked.
5. Remove the pork from the pan and leave to sit for 5 minutes, then shred with a fork.
6. Bring the sauce to the boil, until it has thickened. Mix the pulled pork through the sauce and turn the heat off.
7. Arrange the tortilla chips on a large baking tray and preheat the grill to high. Spoon the pulled pork over the nachos, then top with the cheeses.
8. Grill for 3–4 minutes until the pulled pork is turning slightly crispy and the cheeses have melted. Top with the fresh coriander, sweetcorn and avocado and serve with the lime wedges.

Happier, Healthier, Tastier!

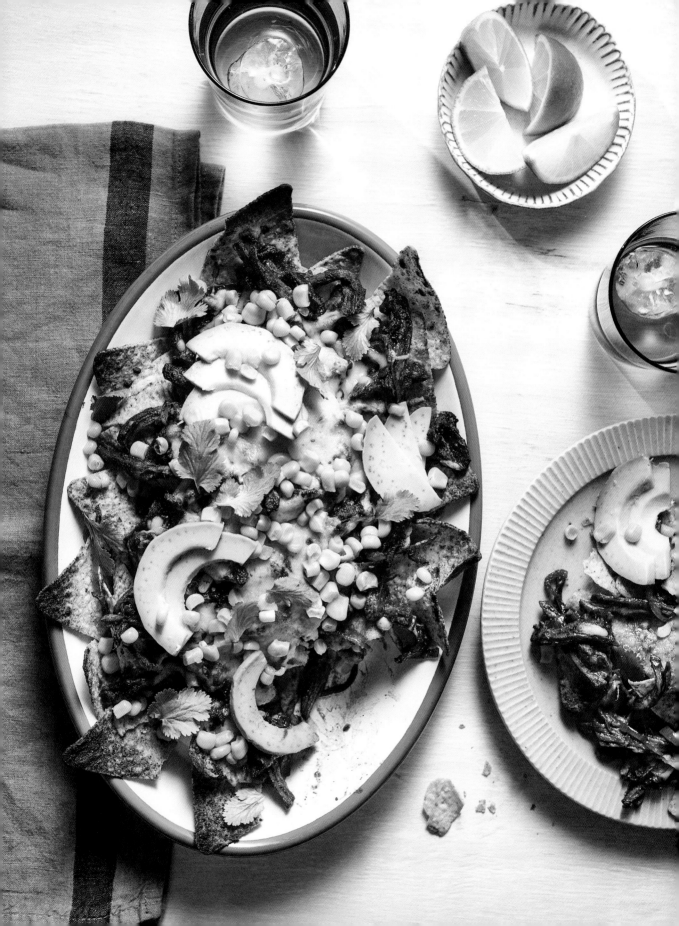

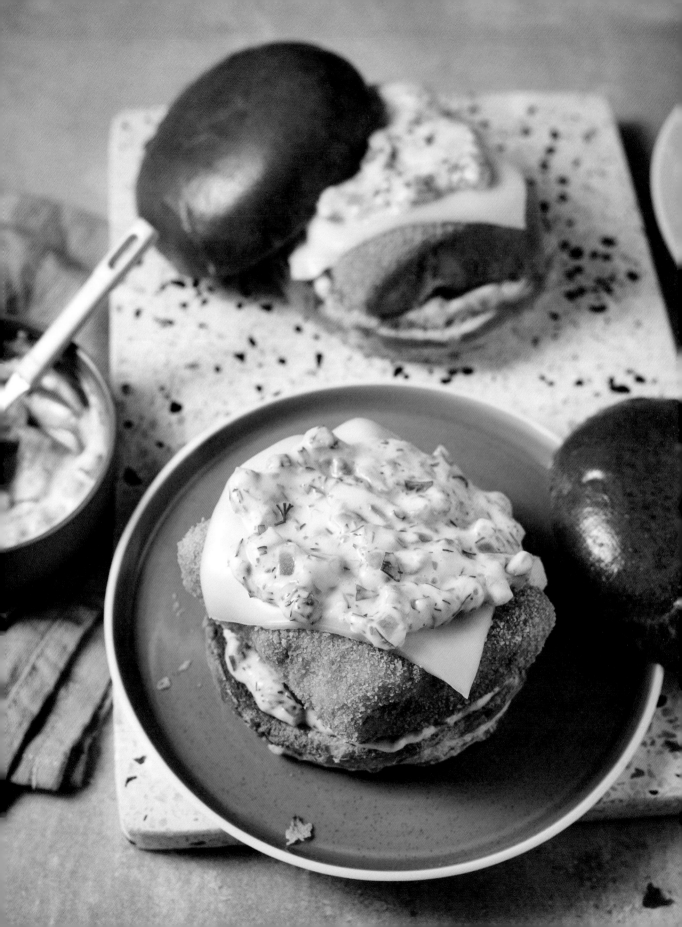

Fish-fillet Burger

Per serving:

Carbs: 29.2g

Calories: 396

Fat: 12g

Protein: 27.9g

Eat your heart out, all you fast-food outlets. My special fish-fillet burger is so much healthier and more delicious than anything you can order in. And it's ready to eat in under thirty minutes, making it a quick and easy supper when you get home from work.

MAKES 2

20g dried golden breadcrumbs
½ tsp garlic powder
½ tsp onion powder
2 cod loins, patted dry
20g plain flour
1 egg, beaten
Low-calorie cooking spray
2 tbsp light mayonnaise
2 pickles, finely chopped
2 tbsp finely chopped capers
2 tsp finely chopped fresh dill
2 tsp finely chopped flat-leaf
  parsley
Juice of 1 lemon
2 brioche burger buns
2 reduced-fat cheese singles
Freshly ground black pepper

1. Preheat the oven to 200°C/180°C Fan/Gas 6.
2. Combine the breadcrumbs, garlic powder and onion powder. Place the flour and the beaten egg in two separate shallow bowls.
3. Dip the cod in the plain flour and dust on all sides, then pat the excess off.
4. Dip the cod in the egg and coat evenly, then dip into the breadcrumb mixture – again, ensuring they are coated evenly.
5. Place on a baking tray and spray with low-calorie cooking spray. Bake in the oven for around 20 minutes, until cooked through and golden.
6. While the cod is roasting, combine the mayonnaise, pickles, capers, dill, parsley, lemon juice and black pepper in a small bowl.
7. Lightly toast the brioche buns, then spoon over half of the sauce, top with the fish and finish with the cheese slices. Spoon over the remaining sauce, top with the brioche bun and serve.

Happier, Healthier, Tastier!

Crispy Pork Souvlaki

Per serving:

Carbs: 39.4g

Calories: 446

Fat: 11g

Protein: 44.4g

Most Greek souvlaki takeaways are very nice, but incredibly naughty with added French fries and a very high calorie count. So why not make them yourself with some easy swaps to turn them into low-cal meals. This is so good that you'll never look back!

SERVES 4
600g lean diced pork
1 tbsp olive oil
1 red pepper, deseeded and sliced into chunks
1 red onion, sliced through the root into wedges (the root will keep them intact)
Juice of 1 lemon
2 tsp dried oregano
1 tsp smoked paprika
1 tsp honey
4 tbsp fat-free yoghurt
4 Greek-style flatbreads
Sea salt
Freshly ground black pepper

1. In a large bowl, combine the pork, olive oil, red pepper, red onion, lemon juice, oregano, smoked paprika and honey. Season well with sea salt and black pepper. Marinate for 10–15 minutes.
2. Preheat the grill to high.
3. Grab some metal skewers and thread the ingredients on, alternating pork, red pepper and red onion.
4. Pop the skewers on a foil-lined baking tray and grill for around 4–5 minutes, then flip and grill for a further 3–4 minutes, until cooked through and deliciously golden.
5. Serve with the yoghurt dolloped over and flatbreads on the side.

Happier, Healthier, Tastier!

Grilled Salmon-loaded Gyros

Per serving:

Carbs: 5.3g

Calories: 492

Fat: 13.7g

Protein: 26.9g

These are probably not only the fastest gyros you'll ever make, but the healthiest, too. Salmon is one of the best sources of protein you can eat, and it's also rich in omega-3 oils that help protect your heart. Mixed with feta, olives and salad in fluffy naans, it's a meal made in heaven.

SERVES 2

1 × 130g skinless salmon fillet
2 tsp smoked paprika
Low-calorie cooking spray
2 mini naans (plain are best)
50g lettuce leaves
30g black olives, pitted and sliced
5 cherry tomatoes, halved
50g reduced-fat feta
2 tbsp light mayonnaise
2 tbsp fat-free yoghurt
Juice of 1 lemon
1 tsp honey
1 tsp dried oregano
Sea salt
Freshly ground black pepper

1. Preheat the grill to medium–high and line a baking tray with non-stick baking paper.
2. Place the salmon fillet on the lined baking tray and sprinkle over the smoked paprika, then spray with cooking spray and season with sea salt and black pepper.
3. Grill the salmon fillet for 4–5 minutes, until lightly golden and cooked through. Flake into large chunks with a knife.
4. Pop the naan breads on a baking tray and grill on both sides for 30 seconds, until heated through.
5. Add the lettuce leaves to the naans, then the salmon chunks.
6. Add the black olives and cherry tomatoes, then crumble over the feta.
7. In a small bowl, mix the mayonnaise, yoghurt, lemon juice, honey and oregano with a fork, then dollop this over the top.
8. Roll up the gyros and enjoy!

Happier, Healthier, Tastier!

Chinese Char Siu Pork with Special Fried Rice

Per serving:

Carbs: 33g

Calories: 476

Fat: 11.2g

Protein: 35.3g

If you order this Cantonese dish as a takeaway it can be very high in calories, but never fear – I have an equally tasty but healthier fakeaway version, made with lean pork fillet. And my special fried rice cooks beautifully with just a few squirts of low-cal spray oil. What's not to like?

SERVES 4

FOR THE CHAR SIU PORK
2 tbsp runny honey
4 tbsp light soy sauce
4 tbsp dark soy sauce
1 tbsp Chinese five-spice
    powder
2 tbsp tomato purée
1 tsp red food colouring
    (optional – for that authentic
    char siu colour)
1 pork tenderloin fillet (about
    500g)
Low-calorie cooking spray

**FOR THE SPECIAL FRIED
RICE**
Low-calorie cooking spray
300g cooked and cooled rice
150g frozen peas
2 eggs, beaten
2 tbsp light soy sauce
6 spring onions, finely sliced

1. Combine the honey, both soy sauces, five-spice powder, tomato purée and red food colouring (if using) in a large dish. Add the pork and rub the ingredients into the meat. It might be a good idea to use plastic gloves to do this, so you don't stain your hands.
2. Now there are two options: you can leave the pork in the fridge overnight, which will make it so much tastier, or you can let it marinate for around an hour in the fridge and cook it straight away.
3. To cook, preheat the oven to 180°C/160°C Fan/Gas 4. Transfer the pork to a foil-lined baking tray and spoon over the marinade. Spray with cooking spray and bake in the oven for 25–30 minutes.
4. To make the special fried rice, spray a large frying pan or wok over a high heat with cooking spray and add the rice. Stir fry for 3–4 minutes, then add the peas and stir-fry for 2 minutes. Add the beaten egg and stir everything well.
5. Stir through the soy sauce and spring onions and serve with the pork.

Happier, Healthier, Tastier!

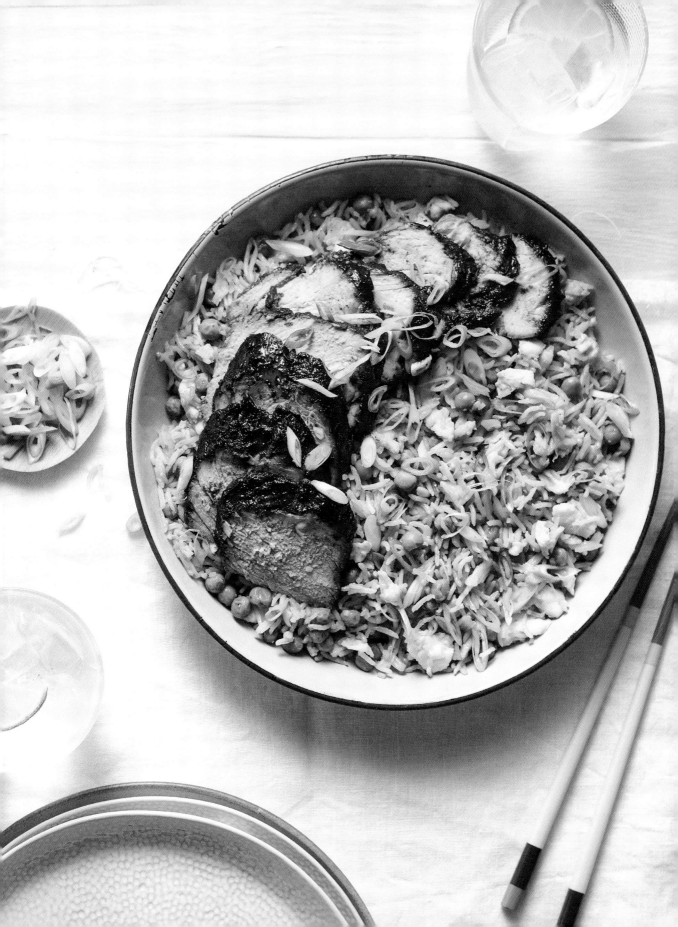

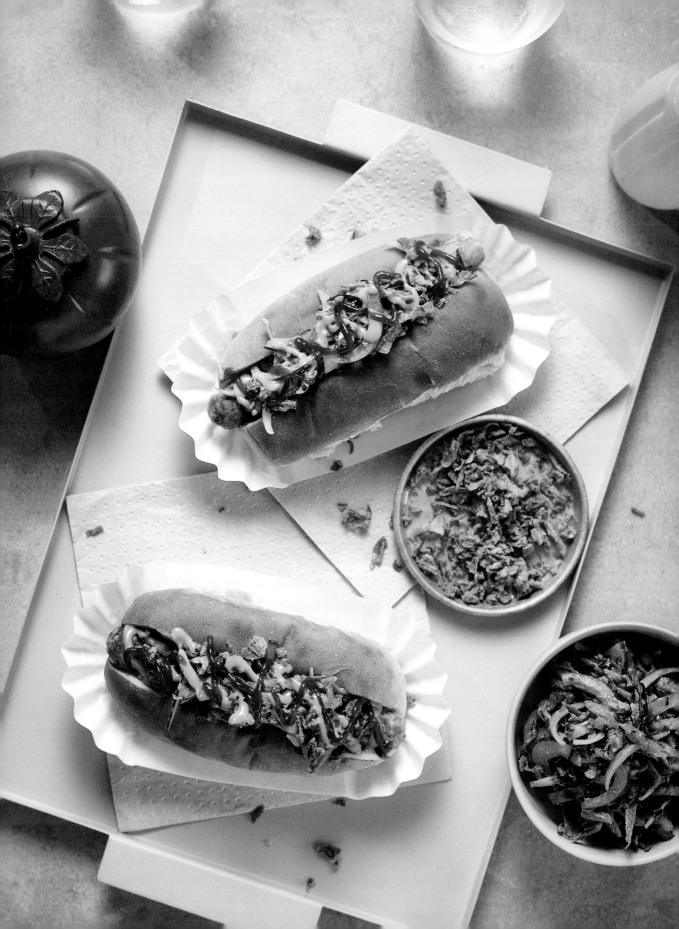

Loaded Hot Dogs

Who doesn't enjoy a hot dog? But many are so high in calories that I decided to tweak the traditional recipe. My healthy take on everyone's favourite fast food is drizzled with ketchup and mustard but uses low-fat chicken sausages and swaps the usual fried onions for a delicious colourful slaw. Try them and you'll be hooked.

Per serving:

Carbs: 52.7g

Calories: 449

Fat: 14.3g

Protein: 28.6g

MAKES 2
4 chicken sausages
1 small carrot, grated
¼ small red cabbage, grated
½ small red onion, very finely sliced
½ apple, grated
1 tbsp fat-free yoghurt
1 tbsp light mayonnaise
2 brioche hot-dog buns
2 tsp shop-bought crispy onions
English mustard and tomato ketchup, to serve
Sea salt
Freshly ground black pepper

1. Preheat the oven to 190°C/170°C Fan/Gas 5 and cook the sausages according to the packet instructions (around 20–25 minutes).
2. Meanwhile, combine the carrot, cabbage, onion, apple, yoghurt and mayonnaise to make the slaw. Season with sea salt and black pepper.
3. Lightly toast the hot-dog buns, then add two sausages per hot dog, top with the slaw and crispy onions, then add a squeeze of mustard and ketchup.

Happier, Healthier, Tastier!

Melt-in-the-middle Fishcakes

Per serving:

Carbs: 35.6g

Calories: 363

Fat: 9.8g

Protein: 32.3g

You can prepare these fishcakes in advance and keep them in the fridge overnight or freeze them to cook at a later date. Baked in the oven, rather than fried, they come with a lovely surprise – when you bite into them, the melted cheese oozes out.

SERVES 4

650g potatoes, peeled and quartered
300g skinless cod
200g frozen peas
1 tbsp wholegrain mustard
10 fresh mint leaves, roughly chopped
2 tbsp capers, roughly chopped
80g reduced-fat Cheddar, cut into 8 cubes
3 slices of bread, blitzed to breadcrumbs
1 tbsp olive oil
100g asparagus, halved
100g Tenderstem broccoli
Lemon wedges, to serve
Sea salt
Freshly ground black pepper

1. Preheat the oven to 200°C/180°C Fan/Gas 6.
2. Add the potatoes to a pan of salted boiling water and boil over a high heat for 13–15 minutes, until cooked through. Add the fish and peas for the final 5 minutes.
3. Remove the fish from the pan and set aside to stream-dry.
4. Drain the potatoes and peas, add the wholegrain mustard, then return to the pan with the mint leaves and capers. Mash together.
5. Carefully add the fish to the mixture by flaking it with your hands into smallish chunks.
6. Divide the cod and potato mixture into 8 balls and, with your finger, push a cube of cheese into the middle of each one. Surround the cheese with the potato mixture, then flatten to create a fishcake shape.
7. Dredge the fishcakes in the breadcrumbs, until they are evenly coated. Heat the olive oil in a medium non-stick frying pan and fry them in batches for 3–4 minutes on each side, until golden.
8. Transfer the fishcakes to a lined baking tray and bake in the oven for 8–10 minutes, until cooked through. You don't want to overcook them, otherwise the cheese will be too cooked to melt.
9. Meanwhile, boil the asparagus and broccoli for 3 minutes, until tender.
10. Serve the fishcakes and vegetables with lemon wedges for squeezing over.

Happier, Healthier, Tastier!

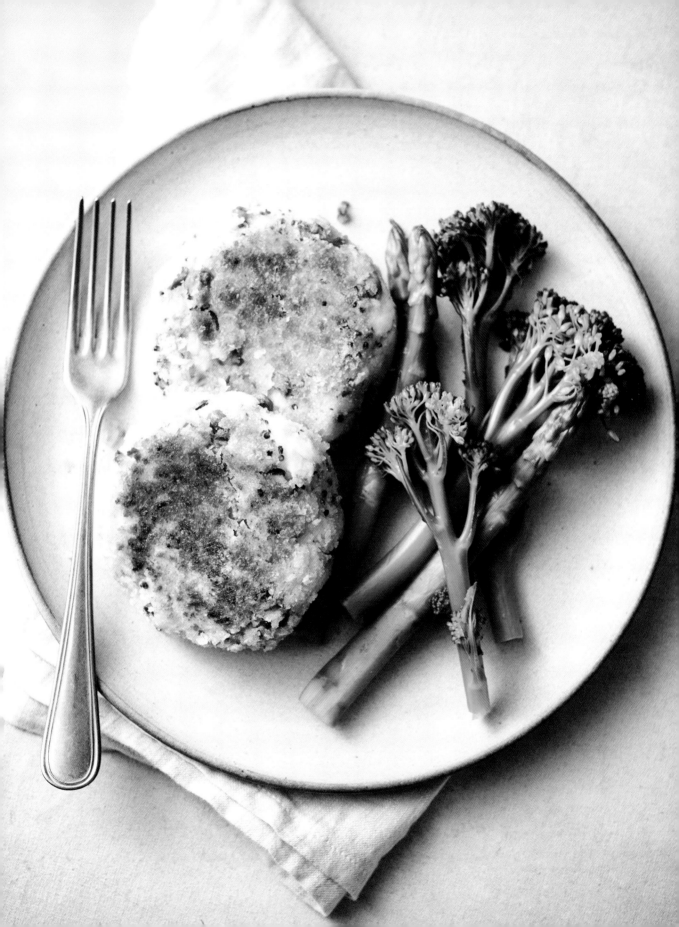

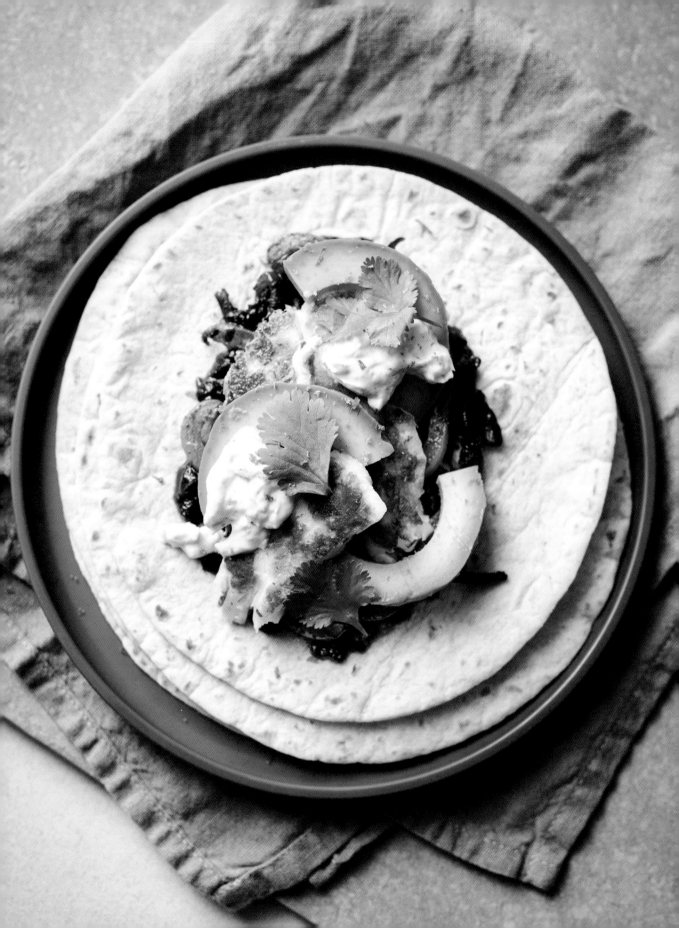

Crispy Halloumi Fajitas ⓥ

Per serving:

Carbs: 40.2g

Calories: 598

Fat: 30.1g

Protein: 37.8g

How insane is this! Not your usual Mexican takeaway, but I love adding crispy golden halloumi to my fajitas. It goes so well with the spicy vegetables, creamy avocado and chilli jam. So go on . . . try it for supper tonight and see how good it is.

SERVES 2

1 tsp olive oil
1 red onion, sliced
1 yellow pepper, deseeded and finely sliced
1 garlic clove, finely chopped
1 heaped tsp smoked paprika
1 tsp ground coriander
Juice and zest of 1 lime
Low-calorie cooking spray
250g reduced-fat halloumi, sliced
2 tsp plain flour
4 mini tortilla wraps
2 tsp chilli jam
1 tbsp light mayonnaise
2 tbsp fat-free yoghurt
½ avocado, sliced
Fresh coriander, to serve
Sea salt
Freshly ground black pepper

1. Heat the olive oil in a non-stick frying pan and fry the red onion and yellow pepper for 4–5 minutes over a medium–high heat, until softened.
2. Add the garlic and fry for a further 1–2 minutes, stirring frequently.
3. Stir through the smoked paprika and ground coriander and fry for a further minute.
4. Squeeze in half of the lime juice and season with sea salt and black pepper.
5. Meanwhile, grab another non-stick frying pan and spray with low-calorie cooking spray over a medium heat. Sprinkle the halloumi pieces with the plain flour and fry in the pan in batches, until golden and crisp all over.
6. Lay out the tortilla wraps and spoon over the chilli jam, then add the onion and pepper mixture.
7. Mix the mayonnaise, yoghurt and the remaining lime juice and zest.
8. Add the crispy halloumi to the wraps, along with the avocado.
9. Dollop over the zesty yoghurt and sprinkle over the fresh coriander, to serve.

Happier, Healthier, Tastier!

Creamy Prawn Laksa

Per serving:

Carbs: 33.3g

Calories: 488

Fat: 26.1g

Protein: 30.8g

This laksa is as good as it gets. It's comfort food at its best and has become one of my favourite winter warmers. Adding coconut milk makes it so wonderfully creamy, while the sugar snap peas and peanuts add crunch. It's heaven in a bowl.

SERVES 2

1 tsp olive oil
1 onion, finely chopped
1 tsp dried chilli flakes
2 garlic cloves, finely chopped
2 tbsp red Thai curry paste
1 × 400g tin light coconut milk
1 tsp fish sauce
400ml vegetable (or fish) stock
100g flat rice noodles
150g sugar snap peas
200g raw king prawns
Juice of 1 lime

TO SERVE

½ bunch of fresh coriander,
   leaves torn
2 tbsp roasted peanuts
Spring onions, finely sliced
1 red chilli, finely sliced

1. Heat the olive oil in a large saucepan over a medium heat and gently fry the onion for 5 minutes, until softened.
2. Add the chilli flakes and garlic and fry for a further 2 minutes, stirring regularly.
3. Add the curry paste and stir it through for 1 minute.
4. Add the coconut milk, fish sauce and stock and bring to the boil.
5. Reduce the heat to medium and add the noodles. Cook for around 3–5 minutes, until softened.
6. Add the sugar snap peas, prawns and lime juice and stir into the sauce. Cook for 3–4 minutes, until the prawns are done and the sugar snap peas are tender but still have a crunch.
7. Serve with torn fresh coriander, roasted peanuts, spring onions and red chilli scattered over.

Happier, Healthier, Tastier!

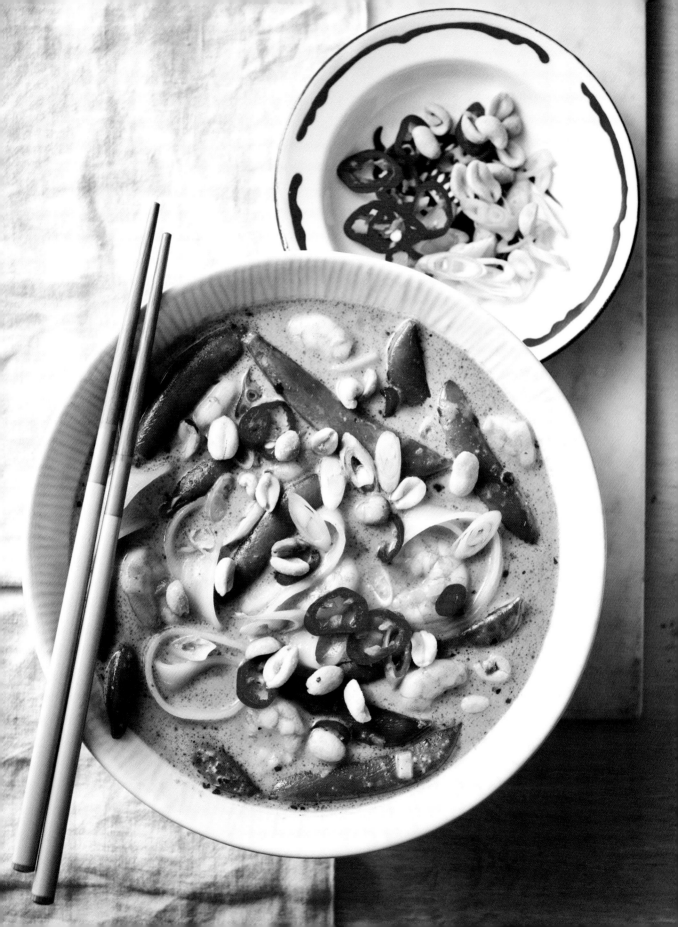

Cheese and Onion Pasties ⓥ

Per serving:

Carbs: 62.7g

Calories: 561

Fat: 26.4g

Protein: 19g

I am a sucker for pasties but so many of the ones you buy are not very healthy, so I've come up with this lighter no-fuss version, which is really easy to make and uses up leftovers, too. To make it even more simple, you can use the ready-rolled light puff-pastry sheets.

MAKES 2
1 tbsp low-fat spread
1 onion, very finely chopped
160g light puff pastry
1 large leftover baked potato
½ tsp Dijon mustard
50g reduced-fat Cheddar, grated
1 egg, beaten
Freshly ground black pepper

1. Preheat the oven to 200°C/180°C Fan/Gas 6.
2. Heat the spread in a small non-stick frying pan over a medium heat, then add the finely chopped onion and fry, stirring frequently, for around 5 minutes, until golden brown and delicious. Leave to cool.
3. Roll out the puff pastry, then cut into four equal rectangles (roughly 10 × 20cm).
4. Slice the baked potato in half and scoop out the flesh into a large bowl. Mash well with a fork, until barely any lumps remain.
5. Stir the cooled onions and Dijon mustard through the mashed potato, then combine with the grated cheese, working the mixture, so it is as smooth as possible. Season with black pepper.
6. Brush the beaten egg around all the edges of the puff-pastry rectangles and add some cheese and potato mixture to two of them, being careful to leave about 2.5cm from the edge clear.
7. Place the remaining pastry rectangles on top and use a fork to seal the two halves together around the edges. Brush some more egg over the top.
8. Bake the pasties in the oven for 15–20 minutes, until golden and puffed up and the cheese has melted.

Happier, Healthier, Tastier!

Tandoori Salmon Burger

Here's a funky twist on the humble burger. Substitute protein-rich, healthy salmon for the beef and flavour with aromatic spices, herbs and ginger. Then serve in soft burger buns, drizzled with cooling cucumber raita. The burgers are so quick and easy to make, but to keep them firm it's a good idea to rest them in the fridge for at least thirty minutes before cooking. A dollop of chilli jam works really nicely in these burgers, too!

Per serving:

Carbs: 31.4g

Calories: 556

Fat: 25.4g

Protein: 47.7g

SERVES 4

4 × 130g boneless, skinless salmon fillets
2 tbsp tandoori paste
½ bunch fresh coriander, roughly chopped
1 garlic clove, roughly chopped
Thumb-sized piece of ginger, roughly chopped
1 egg, beaten
1 tsp plain flour
2 tbsp olive oil
4 tbsp fat-free yoghurt
¼ cucumber, grated
Juice of ½ lemon
4 brioche burger buns
1 carrot, peeled and cut into ribbons with a speed peeler
1 red onion, finely sliced
Sea salt
Freshly ground black pepper

1. Place the salmon fillets, tandoori paste, coriander, garlic, ginger and egg in a food processor and pulse until roughly minced. Season with sea salt and black pepper.
2. Shape the mixture into four burger patties and sprinkle over a dusting of plain flour. If you've got time, pop the patties in the fridge for 30 minutes to firm up. You don't need to do this, but it'll help to prevent them from falling apart when frying.
3. Heat the olive oil in a large non-stick frying pan and fry the burgers for 5 minutes on each side over a medium heat, until crisp and cooked through.
4. In a small bowl, mix the yoghurt, cucumber and lemon juice and season with some more sea salt and black pepper.
5. Load your burgers by spooning the delicious cucumber yoghurt over the brioche bases, then top with the salmon patties, then the carrot ribbons and sliced red onion. Finish with the brioche tops.

Happier, Healthier, Tastier!

Meal Prep Lunches

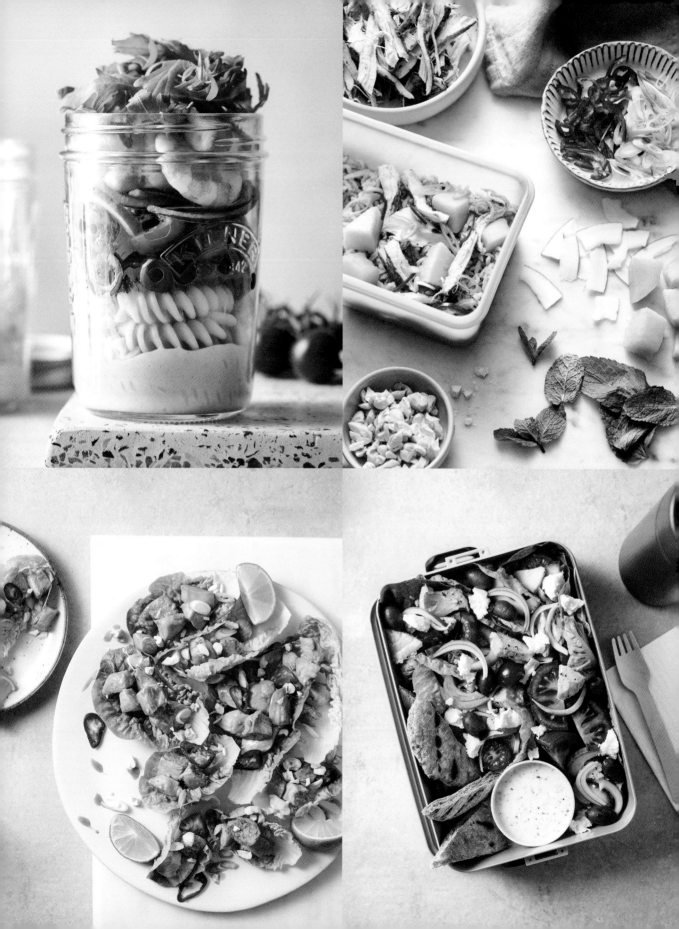

Mason-jar Pasta Salad
Mediterranean Sausage
and Roasted Vegetables
Taco Bowls
Sausage and Kale Gnocchi
Bolognese Risotto
Thai Roasted Chicken and Mango Box
Greek Salmon Salad
Chili con Pasta Bake
Spanish Tortilla
Chicken Pesto Pasta
Bang Bang Chicken Noodle Salad
Teriyaki Chicken Lettuce Wraps
Chicken and Avocado Burritos
Chicken and Chorizo Rice

Mason-jar Pasta Salad

Mason (or Kilner) jars are so useful – not only for making preserves and pickles, but also for layering up salads that you can prepare the night before and take to work with you the following day. The most important thing for a Mason jar salad to work is to keep the dressing at the bottom of the jar – this way the salad won't go soggy as that stays at the top.

Per jar:

Carbs: 62.7g

Calories: 439

Fat: 10.2g

Protein: 27g

MAKES 4 JARS

300g dried pasta (fusilli/ farfalle/penne)
2 tbsp olive oil
2 tsp Dijon mustard
2 tsp honey
1 tbsp apple cider vinegar
Juice of ½ lemon
4 tbsp black olives, pitted
16 cherry tomatoes, halved
½ large red onion, very finely sliced
300g king prawns, cooked and peeled
4 handfuls of fresh rocket leaves
Sea salt
Freshly ground black pepper

1. Cook the pasta in salted, boiling water, according to the packet instructions. Drain and set aside.
2. Whisk together the olive oil, Dijon mustard, honey, apple cider vinegar, lemon juice and a good sprinkling of sea salt and black pepper, until combined. Pour a small amount into the bottom of four Mason jars.
3. Divide the pasta between the jars, then top with some olives, cherry tomatoes and red onion, then the prawns and the rocket on top.
4. To serve, simply give the Mason jar a shake, or empty it out on to a plate. These jar salads will keep in the fridge for 2–4 days.

Happier, Healthier, Tastier!

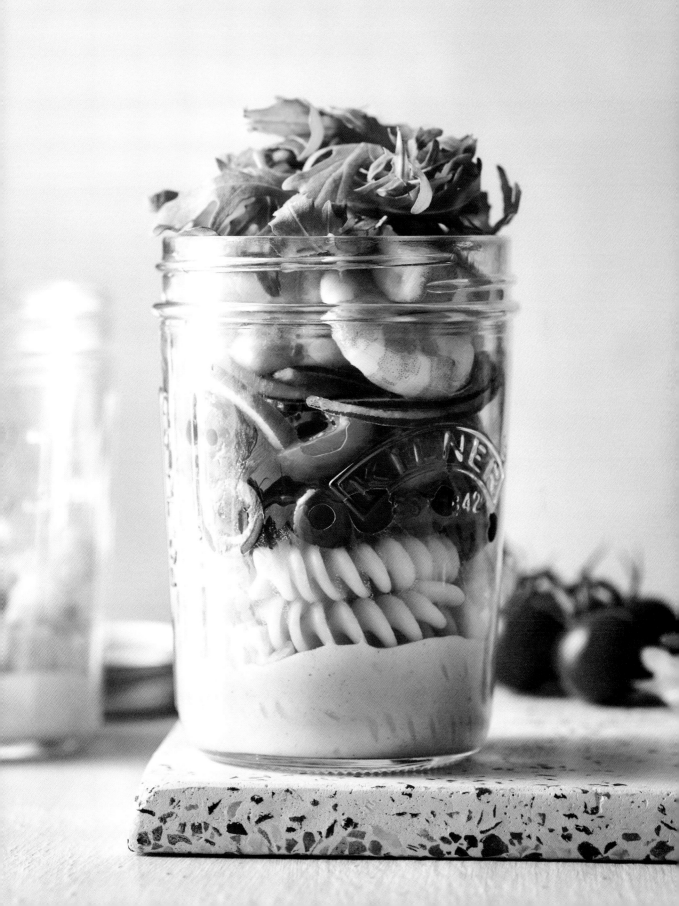

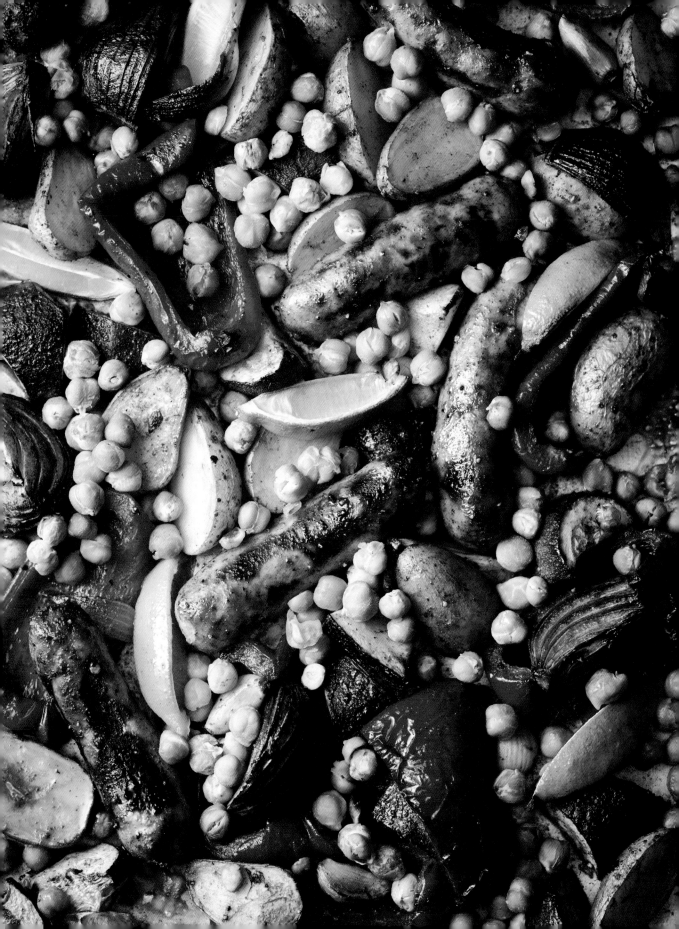

Mediterranean Sausage and Roasted Vegetables

Per serving:

Carbs: 45.9g

Calories: 380

Fat: 8.3g

Protein: 28.1g

This takes a little while to cook, but you can prep all the vegetables in advance and then just arrange them in a roasting pan with the sausages and flavourings. Pop them in the oven and sit back and relax while they roast to crisp perfection. Sheer bliss!

SERVES 4

8 reduced-fat pork sausages
300g miniature new potatoes, halved
2 red peppers, deseeded and quartered
2 red onions, quartered
1 courgette, cut into large chunks
4 garlic cloves, left whole
1 tbsp olive oil
1 tbsp maple syrup
1 tbsp smoked paprika
2 sprigs of thyme
1 × 400g tin chickpeas, drained
1 lemon, cut into wedges
Sea salt
Freshly ground black pepper

1. Preheat the oven to 200°C/180°C Fan/Gas 6.
2. Place the sausages, potatoes, red peppers, red onions, courgette and garlic in a large roasting tray.
3. In a bowl, whisk the olive oil, maple syrup, smoked paprika, thyme sprigs and some sea salt and black pepper and pour over the sausages and vegetables. Stir to ensure everything is well coated. Cover tightly with foil and bake in the oven for around 25–30 minutes.
4. Remove from the oven and stir through the chickpeas. Nestle the lemon wedges in and around the vegetables and return to the oven, without the foil, for a further 30 minutes, until the sausages are cooked and the potatoes are tender.

Happier, Healthier, Tastier!

Taco Bowls

These taco bowls taste as good as they look. If you're busy, you can even cook the beef mince ahead of time to reheat with some leftover rice if you've got some, plus prep the sweetcorn salsa and keep it covered in the fridge, until you're ready to assemble and serve the tacos. You could also assemble the taco bowls into containers ready for lunches.

Per serving:

Carbs: 49g

Calories: 402

Fat: 20g

Protein: 27.6g

SERVES 2

100g sweetcorn
60g cherry tomatoes, halved
3 spring onions, finely sliced
2 tbsp fresh coriander, finely chopped
Juice of ½ lime
2 tsp olive oil
1 red onion, finely sliced
1 red pepper, deseeded and finely sliced
1 garlic clove, finely chopped
150g lean beef mince
1 tbsp fajita mix
120ml tomato passata
½ tbsp sriracha sauce
140g brown rice
½ x 400g tin black beans, drained
Sea salt
Freshly ground black pepper

1. Make the sweetcorn salsa by combining the sweetcorn, tomatoes, spring onions, coriander and lime juice. Set aside.
2. Heat 1 teaspoon of the olive oil in a large non-stick frying pan and fry the red onion and red pepper for 5 minutes, until softened, then stir through the garlic and fry for a further minute.
3. Add the beef mince, breaking up with a wooden spoon, and cook for 5 minutes, until browned.
4. Stir in the fajita mix, then add the tomato passata and sriracha and season with sea salt and black pepper. Leave to gently bubble for 5 minutes, until slightly thickened.
5. Cook the brown rice according to the packet instructions. Drain and combine with the black beans.
6. Serve the beans and rice with the beef mix and sweetcorn salsa.

Happier, Healthier, Tastier!

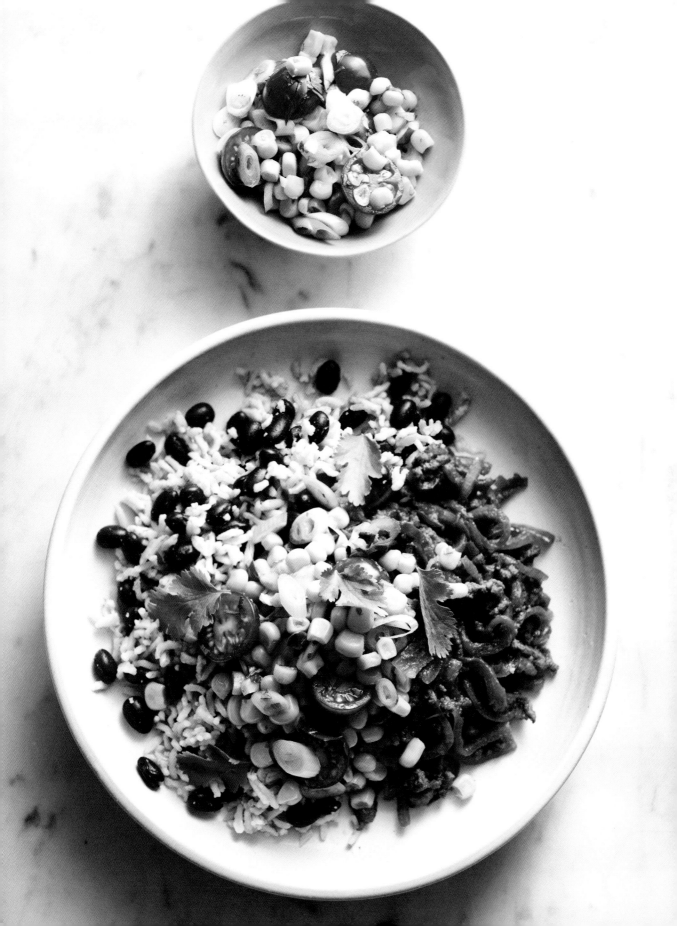

Sausage and Kale Gnocchi

Per serving:

Carbs: 46g

Calories: 390

Fat: 13.3g

Protein: 20.2g

A packet of deli or supermarket gnocchi makes a quick and easy lunch and this dish is perfect for prepping ahead of time. I like to add some homely sausage meat, healthy kale, hot chilli and fennel seeds and a finishing touch of Parmesan.

SERVES 4

1 tbsp olive oil
6 reduced-fat pork sausages, meat squeezed out of the skins
1 onion, finely chopped
2 tsp fennel seeds
½ tsp dried chilli flakes
450ml chicken stock
100g kale, thick stalks removed
450g gnocchi
40g Parmesan, grated
Zest of 1 lemon
Freshly ground black pepper

1. Heat the olive oil in a large non-stick frying pan over a medium heat and, when hot, crumble in the sausage meat, breaking it apart with a wooden spoon. Fry for 5 minutes, stirring frequently.
2. Add the onion, fennel seeds and chilli flakes and fry for a further 4–5 minutes, until the onions have softened.
3. Pour in the chicken stock and simmer, until reduced slightly. Add the kale for 3 minutes, until tender.
4. Cook the gnocchi in boiling water and, once they have risen to the surface, drain and add to the pan with the sausage.
5. Top with the grated Parmesan, lemon zest and a good sprinkling of black pepper.

Happier, Healthier, Tastier!

Bolognese Risotto

Bet you never thought of this before! I enjoy experimenting with different ingredients and flavours and, even though it may sound odd, swapping pasta for rice in your Bolognese sauce is a real winner. So give it a go and see for yourself how tasty it is. This dish can be easily portioned into containers so that you have delicious lunches on hand if you have a busy week coming up.

Per serving:

Carbs: 49.8g

Calories: 369

Fat: 18.2g

Protein: 25g

SERVES 4

1 tbsp olive oil
1 onion, finely diced
1 carrot, finely diced
3 garlic cloves, finely grated
300g lean beef mince
200g risotto rice
1 tbsp tomato purée
400g tomato passata
1 tsp honey
1 tsp Italian herbs
1 litre beef stock
4 tbsp grated Parmesan
½ bunch fresh basil, torn
Sea salt
Freshly ground black pepper

1. Grab a large non-stick frying pan and heat the olive oil. Fry the onion, carrot and garlic over a medium heat for 3–4 minutes, until softened.
2. Add the beef and break up with a wooden spoon, frying until browned all over. This should take about 8 minutes, as you want some decent colour on the beef. Colour = flavour.
3. Stir in the risotto rice and keep stirring for 1–2 minutes.
4. Add the tomato purée and stir it through the mince and vegetables.
5. Add the passata, honey and Italian herbs and season well with sea salt and black pepper.
6. Add the beef stock, 100ml at a time, stirring constantly. Only add more stock once the previous addition has been absorbed. Repeat until you've used all the stock. This will probably take about 20 minutes.
7. Pop a lid on the pan, turn the heat off and let the risotto sit for 5 minutes.
8. When you're ready to serve, sprinkle over the Parmesan and fresh basil.

Happier, Healthier, Tastier!

Thai Roasted Chicken and Mango Box

Per serving:

Carbs: 68.2g

Calories: 408

Fat: 5.3g

Protein: 49g

An easy-peasy lunch box, and so delicious. You can prepare it all in advance the evening before and, when it's cool, pop it into a sealed container and store overnight in the fridge. This recipe makes four portions, so there's enough for several days or for supper as well.

SERVES 4

1 tbsp seven-spice Thai seasoning

4 boneless, skinless chicken breasts

Juice of 1½ limes

200g brown basmati rice

300g mango chunks

1 tbsp flaked coconut

1 bunch of spring onions, trimmed and finely sliced

1 red chilli, deseeded and finely sliced

2 tbsp cashew nuts, chopped

½ bunch of fresh mint, roughly chopped

1. Preheat the oven to 200°C/180°C Fan/Gas 6.
2. Rub the seasoning into the chicken and squeeze over the juice of half a lime. Place on a baking tray and bake for around 20–25 minutes, until it is cooked through, no pink remains and the juices run clear.
3. Meanwhile, cook the brown rice according to the packet instructions, then drain.
4. Roughly shred the chicken and then mix with the mango and rice.
5. Mix through the remaining lime juice, the coconut and spring onions, then sprinkle over the chilli, cashew nuts and fresh mint.

Happier, Healthier, Tastier!

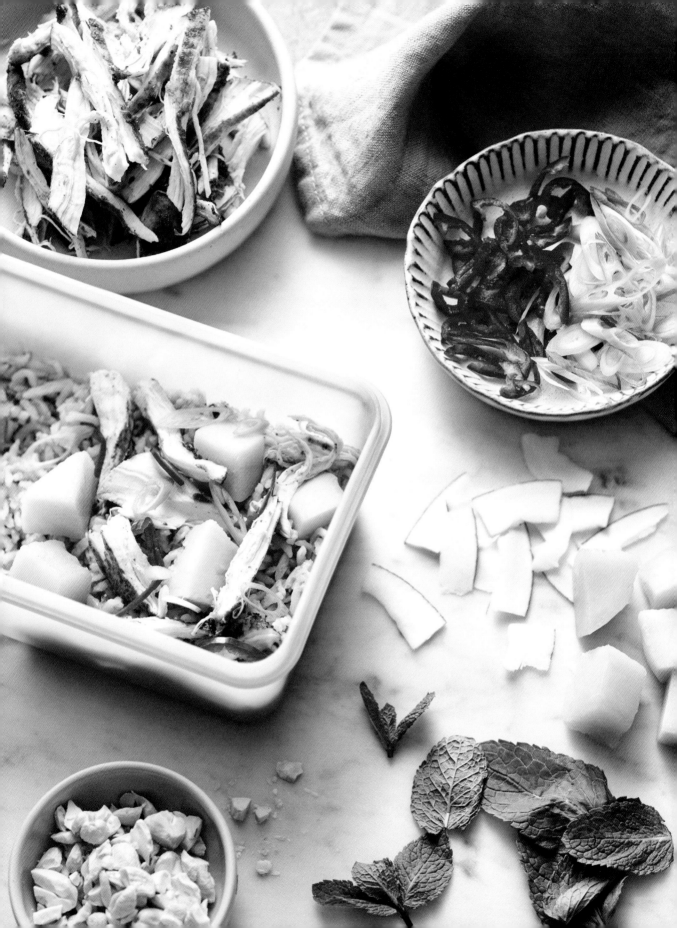

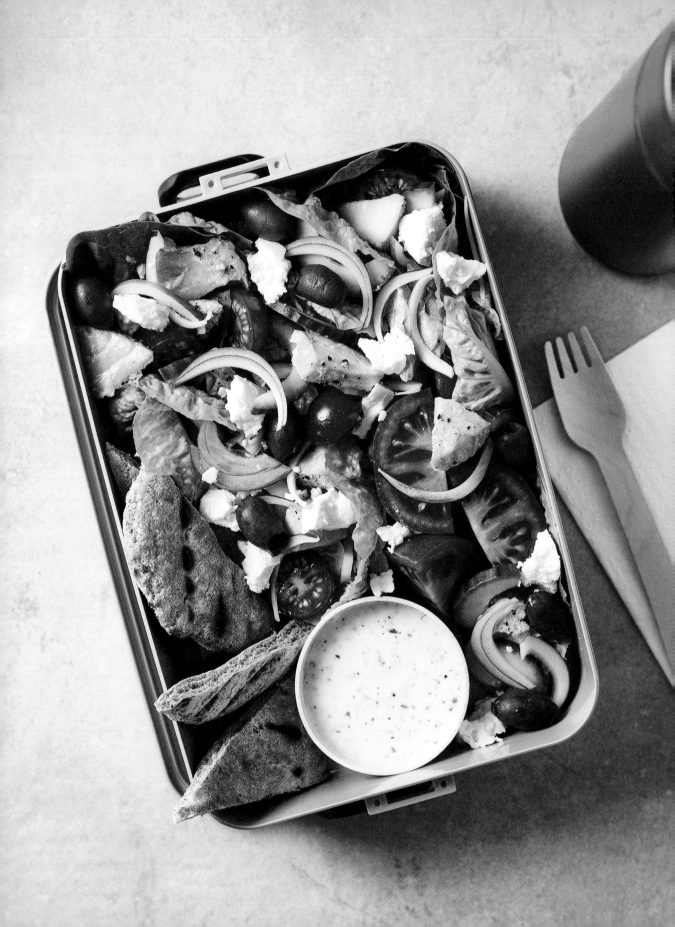

Greek Salmon Salad

Per serving:

Carbs: 49.1g

Calories: 584

Fat: 33.1g

Protein: 34.1g

A prep-ahead meal doesn't come quicker or healthier than this one – and you get a whacking hit of protein, too. Pitta breads are great for splitting and filling with salad, whether for a packed lunch or a relaxed supper.

SERVES 4

4 × 130g salmon fillets
Low-calorie cooking spray
1 cucumber, sliced in half lengthways, deseeded, then sliced into cubes
20 pitted black olives
4 Little Gem lettuces
4 vine tomatoes, quartered
20 cherry tomatoes, halved
1 red onion, finely sliced
2 tbsp olive oil
2 tbsp apple cider vinegar
1 tsp honey
1 tbsp fat-free yoghurt
½ garlic clove, finely grated
1 tsp dried oregano
80g reduced-fat feta, crumbled
4 pitta breads
Sea salt
Freshly ground black pepper

1. Heat the grill to medium–high and spray the salmon with low-calorie cooking spray, then season with sea salt and black pepper.
2. Grill the salmon on a baking tray, skin-side down, for 4–5 minutes, until cooked through and golden.
3. While the salmon is grilling, arrange the cucumber, olives, lettuce, tomatoes and onion in meal-prep boxes.
4. Whisk together the olive oil, apple cider vinegar, honey, fat-free yoghurt, garlic and dried oregano. Keep the dressing in a separate container, so it doesn't make your salad soggy in the fridge. Then simply mix it through the salad when you're ready to eat, along with the crumbled feta.
5. Remove the salmon from the grill, then grill the pitta breads for 40–60 seconds on each side until puffed up and golden. Slice into long triangles and keep separate for when you're ready to eat your prepared lunch.

Happier, Healthier, Tastier!

Chili con Pasta Bake

Sometimes it's fun to be adventurous and ring the changes. You don't have to always eat chili con carne with rice – it's great with pasta, too. Just boil your favourite pasta shapes while the chili's cooking, then tip everything into an ovenproof dish, sprinkle with cheese and bake until golden brown, bubbling and crispy. This can then be portioned into containers for easy lunches.

Per serving:

Carbs: 30.8g

Calories: 409

Fat: 27.9g

Protein: 40.1g

SERVES 4

1 tbsp olive oil
1 onion, finely chopped
1 red pepper, deseeded and chopped
2 garlic cloves, finely grated
500g lean beef mince
1 tsp ground cumin
2 tsp mild chilli powder
1 × 400g tin chopped tomatoes
1 tsp honey
1 × 400g tin kidney beans, drained
250ml beef stock
300g dried pasta (such as penne)
40g reduced-fat cheese, grated
40g reduced-fat mozzarella, grated
Sea salt
Freshly ground black pepper

1. Preheat the oven to 200°C/180°C Fan/Gas 6.
2. Heat the olive oil in a large non-stick frying pan and fry the onion and pepper for 5 minutes, until softened.
3. Stir in the garlic and fry for 1 minute.
4. Add the beef mince, breaking up with the back of a spoon, and cook for around 5 minutes, until browned.
5. Sprinkle over the spices and stir for 1 minute.
6. Add the chopped tomatoes, honey, kidney beans and beef stock and bring to the boil. Season well with sea salt and black pepper. Reduce the heat and simmer for 15 minutes while you cook the pasta.
7. Boil the pasta according to the packet instructions, then drain and stir into the chili.
8. Transfer to a baking dish and top with the cheeses.
9. Bake in the oven for around 20 minutes, until golden.

Happier, Healthier, Tastier!

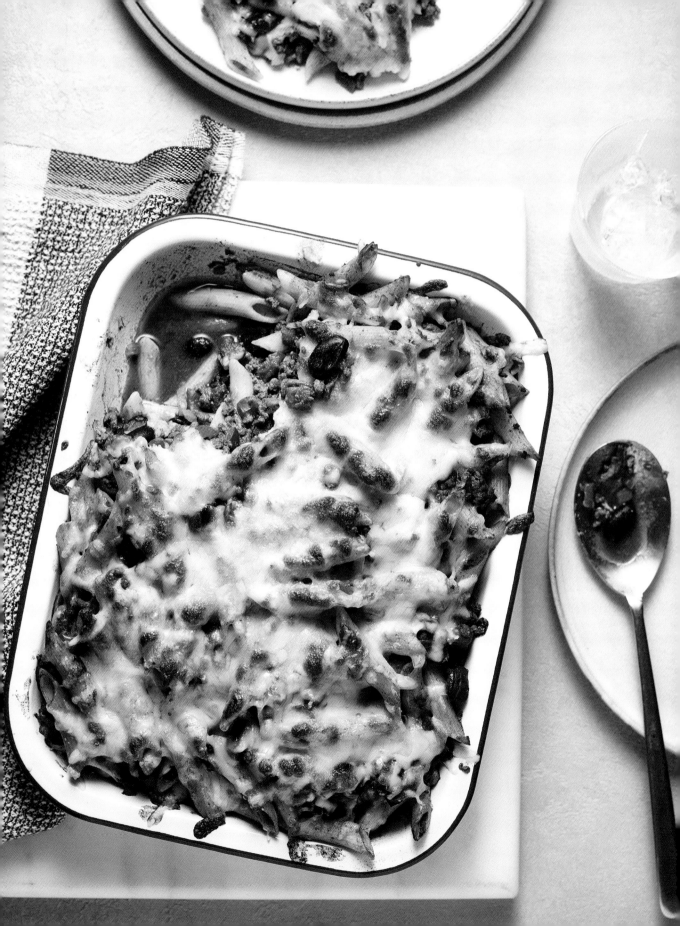

Spanish Tortilla 🅥

Here's my take on the classic tortilla. And it's not just the fantastic flavours that make it so special – it's really low in calories, too, and packed with protein. To speed it up, you can use leftover boiled potatoes, rather than cooking them from scratch. A good Monday lunchtime treat or supper to follow the Sunday roast.

Per serving:

Carbs: 25.6g

Calories: 327

Fat: 15.8g

Protein: 20.8g

SERVES 4

700g potatoes, peeled and
   very finely sliced
1 tsp olive oil
1 onion, very finely sliced
65g diced chorizo
2 garlic cloves, finely chopped
6 large eggs, beaten
40g reduced-fat Cheddar,
   grated
Sea salt
Freshly ground black pepper

1. Cook the potatoes in salted boiling water over a high heat for 3 minutes, then drain well and leave to steam- dry.
2. Meanwhile, heat the olive oil in a large non-stick, ovenproof frying pan and fry the onion and chorizo, until the chorizo releases its lovely golden oil and the onion is softened (around 5 minutes).
3. Add the garlic and fry for a further 2 minutes.
4. Add the potatoes to the pan and give everything a good mix to coat them.
5. Roughly arrange the potatoes, so they are distributed evenly around the pan and layered on top of each other.
6. Pour the eggs over the mixture and reduce the heat to low. Gently cook for 15–20 minutes, until the mixture has set.
7. Turn the grill to high, sprinkle the cheese over your tortilla and pop the pan under the grill for 3–4 minutes, until the top has browned, then season with black pepper. Serve with a simple salad.

Happier, Healthier, Tastier!

Chicken Pesto Pasta

Pasta is always a firm family favourite. It's become the world's best-loved food and no wonder – there are so many types and shapes and it's infinitely versatile. You can use any of your preferred pasta shapes in this yummy dish. I love to serve it with a tasty salad of rocket and pine nuts, drizzled with a sweet balsamic glaze. It's perfect for lunches on-the-go.

Per serving:

Carbs: 59.8g

Calories: 544

Fat: 19g

Protein: 35.8g

SERVES 4

300g short pasta (farfalle, penne, etc.)
1 head of broccoli, cut into florets
1 tbsp olive oil
1 small onion, finely chopped
2 skinless, boneless chicken breasts (cut into strips)
4 tbsp pesto (green or red)
2 tbsp pine nuts
30g Parmesan, grated
16 mini mozzarella balls
2 large handfuls of rocket leaves
Balsamic glaze, to serve
Sea salt
Freshly ground black pepper

1. Cook the pasta according to the packet instructions, adding the broccoli florets for the final 2 minutes. Drain, reserving a little pasta water, and set aside.
2. Meanwhile, heat the olive oil in a large non-stick frying pan and fry the onion over a medium heat for 3–4 minutes, then add the chicken and fry for a further 6–8 minutes, until cooked through and golden. Season everything with sea salt and black pepper.
3. Add the pesto and stir through with a splash of the pasta water.
4. Add the drained pasta and broccoli to the pan and give everything a good toss to combine.
5. Serve with the pine nuts scattered over, along with the grated Parmesan, mozzarella balls and rocket leaves.
6. Drizzle the salad with a nice drop of balsamic glaze.

Happier, Healthier, Tastier!

Bang Bang Chicken Noodle Salad

Per serving:

Carbs: 34.4g

Calories: 337

Fat: 9.8g

Protein: 27.4g

There may be a long list of ingredients here, but don't let that put you off. This is one of the best meals you'll ever eat and could become your signature dish. So stop whatever you're doing right now, write that shopping list and get down to the supermarket. It really is sublime!

SERVES 4

2 boneless, skinless chicken breasts
2 tsp Chinese five-spice powder
100g medium egg noodles
150g frozen peas
1 tsp toasted sesame oil
1 courgette, spiralised
3 carrots, peeled and spiralised
3 spring onions, finely sliced
1 red chilli, deseeded and finely sliced
1 tbsp almond butter (or peanut butter)
3 tbsp soy sauce
1 tbsp honey
Juice of 1 lime
½ garlic clove, finely grated
1 tsp sesame seeds
40g roasted peanuts
½ bunch of fresh coriander, roughly chopped
Sea salt
Freshly ground black pepper

1. Preheat the oven to 200°C/180°C Fan/Gas 6.
2. Place the chicken breasts on a lined baking tray, season with salt and pepper and sprinkle over the five-spice powder. Bake for 25–30 minutes, until completely cooked through. Leave to cool, then shred with two forks.
3. Cook the noodles for 3–5 minutes or according to the packet instructions, adding the peas for the final minute. Drain and toss in the sesame oil to stop them sticking together. Leave to cool.
4. Add the courgette, carrots, spring onions and red chilli to a large bowl, then stir through the cooled noodles, peas and shredded chicken.
5. In a small bowl, whisk the almond butter with a splash of kettle water, until loosened. Then stir through the soy sauce, honey, lime juice and garlic, until combined. Pour over the salad.
6. Sprinkle the sesame seeds, roasted peanuts and fresh coriander over the top, to serve.

Happier, Healthier, Tastier!

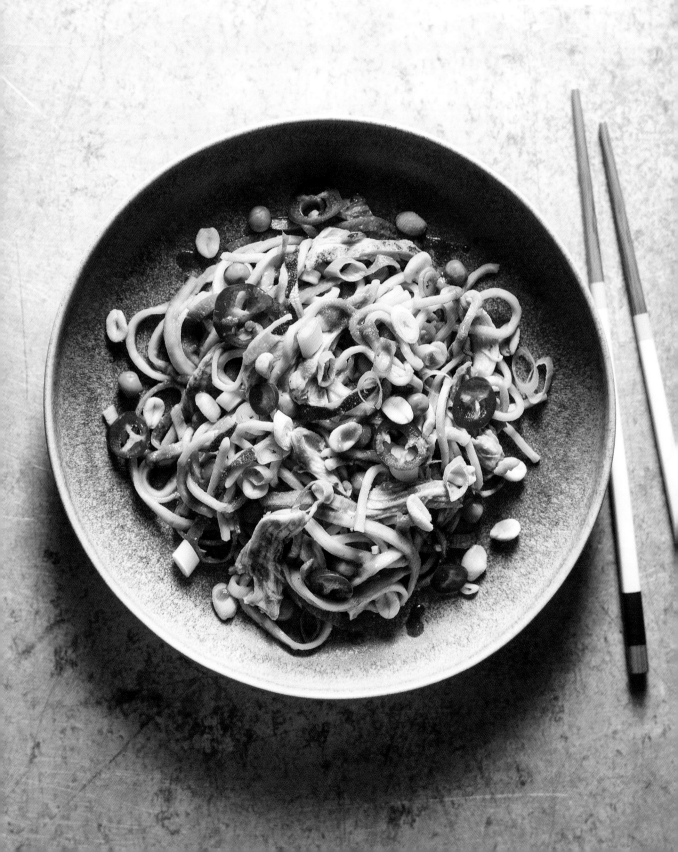

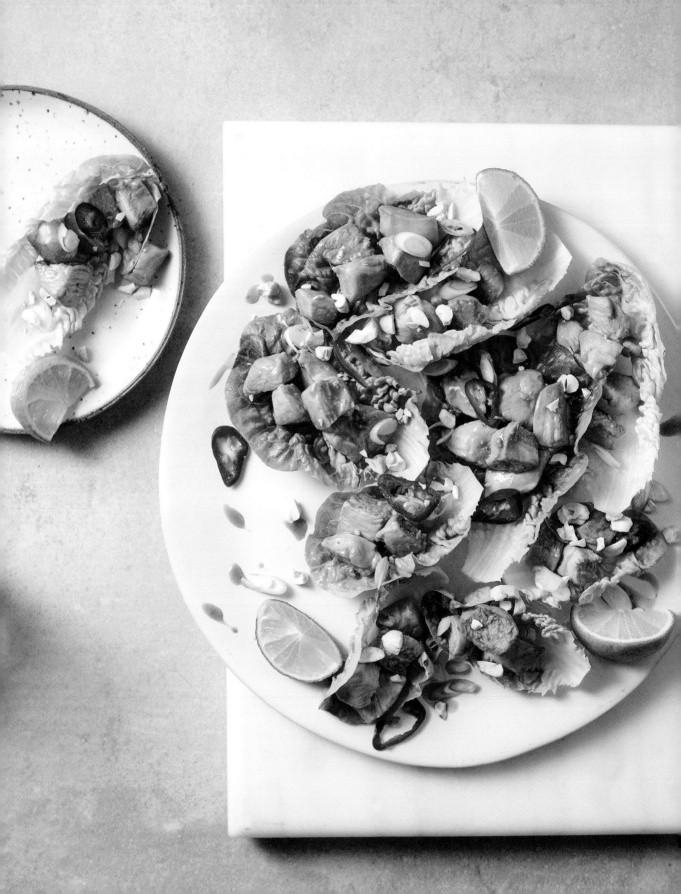

Teriyaki Chicken Lettuce Wraps

Per serving:

Carbs: 49.4g

Calories: 257

Fat: 7.1g

Protein: 55.4g

I sometimes use crisp lettuce leaves instead of tortillas or flatbreads to make really healthy wraps. They're low-carb, low-fat and a sprinkling of cashews makes them refreshingly crunchy. If you prefer, you could substitute turkey breast meat for the chicken. Pack the chicken and toppings separately to the lettuce leaves to keep the lettuce crisp for an easy to assemble packed lunch.

SERVES 2

1 tsp olive oil
2 boneless, skinless chicken
   breasts, cut into small cubes
1 tsp honey
2 tbsp teriyaki sauce
1 garlic clove, finely grated
1 tbsp dark soy sauce
1 tsp cornflour
Juice of 2 limes
1–2 Little Gem lettuces, ends
   removed and large leaves
   reserved
1 red chilli, deseeded and
   finely sliced
2 tbsp cashew nuts, roughly
   chopped
2 spring onions, finely sliced

1. Heat the olive oil in a large non-stick frying pan and fry the chicken until browned all over and cooked through (around 5 minutes), stirring regularly.
2. In a small bowl, mix the honey, teriyaki sauce, garlic, soy sauce, cornflour and the juice of 1 lime, until well combined. Pour over the chicken and stir to coat it in the sauce. Leave to bubble for a couple of minutes, until thickened.
3. Load the chicken mixture into the lettuce 'cups' and top with the red chilli, cashew nuts and spring onions. Squeeze over the remaining lime juice.

Happier, Healthier, Tastier!

Chicken and Avocado Burritos

Per serving:

Carbs: 44g

Calories: 473

Fat: 17.1g

Protein: 31.6g

These fabulous, healthy burritos are so dreamy and delicious, and you don't have to worry about the calories. Just cook and assemble them, and wrap them in foil or beeswax wraps ready to take for lunch the next day.

MAKES 4

2 boneless, skinless chicken breasts
1 tbsp olive oil
1 red onion, finely sliced
1 red pepper, deseeded and finely sliced
1 tbsp smoked paprika
1 × 400g tin black beans, drained
100g spinach
2 × 250g pouches of ready-cooked lime and coriander rice
4 tbsp fat-free yoghurt
4 tortilla wraps
1 avocado, mashed
80g reduced-fat Cheddar, grated
Sea salt
Freshly ground black pepper

1. Preheat the oven to 220°C/200°C Fan/Gas 7. Place the chicken breasts on a foil-lined baking tray, season with sea salt and black pepper and bake in the oven for 20–25 minutes, until cooked through and no pink remains.
2. Meanwhile, heat the olive oil in a medium non-stick frying pan over a medium heat and fry the red onion and red pepper for 5 minutes, until softened.
3. Sprinkle over the smoked paprika and stir well, frying for a further 2 minutes. Season well with sea salt and black pepper.
4. Add the black beans to the pan, along with the spinach, and let the spinach wilt.
5. Meanwhile, cook the rice in the microwave, according to the packet instructions.
6. When the chicken is cooked, remove from the oven and, once cool enough to handle, shred roughly with a fork.
7. To assemble the burritos, spoon some yoghurt around the base of each tortilla wrap, then divide the rice between them.
8. Top with the mashed avocado, then the grated cheese, then the shredded chicken and, finally, the vegetables and black beans. Fold the wrap around the fillings and enjoy.

Happier, Healthier, Tastier!

Chicken and Chorizo Rice

Remember those summer holidays in Spain when a large pan of colourful paella arrived at your table and everyone got stuck in? Well, this is the fast-food equivalent that you can rustle up at home, with spicy chorizo, roasted red peppers and smoky paprika. It's the perfect one-pan meal that can easily be portioned into containers ready to tuck into for lunch the next day.

Per serving:

Carbs: 34.7g

Calories: 582

Fat: 33.1g

Protein: 37g

SERVES 4

1 tbsp olive oil
1 onion, finely chopped
2 garlic cloves, finely chopped
2 roasted red peppers, from a jar
6 boneless, skinless chicken thighs, cut into small chunks
100g diced chorizo
1 tsp smoked paprika
1 tbsp tomato purée
500ml chicken stock
300g long-grain rice
100g frozen peas
2 tbsp fresh flat-leaf parsley, to serve
Sea salt
Freshly ground black pepper

1. Heat the olive oil in a large non-stick frying pan over a medium heat and add the onion. Fry for 4–5 minutes, then add the garlic and fry for a further minute.
2. Add the roasted red peppers and stir them through.
3. Increase the heat slightly and add the chicken chunks, diced chorizo and smoked paprika. Fry for around 5 minutes.
4. Stir through the tomato purée and cook for 1 minute.
5. Add the chicken stock and rice and bring to the boil. Season with sea salt and black pepper, then reduce the heat to low and simmer for 15–20 minutes, covered, until all the water has been absorbed by the rice.
6. Stir through the frozen peas, replace the lid and cook, until the peas are done (around 3 minutes).
7. Serve, scattered with parsley.

Happier, Healthier, Tastier!

Vegetarian & Vegan

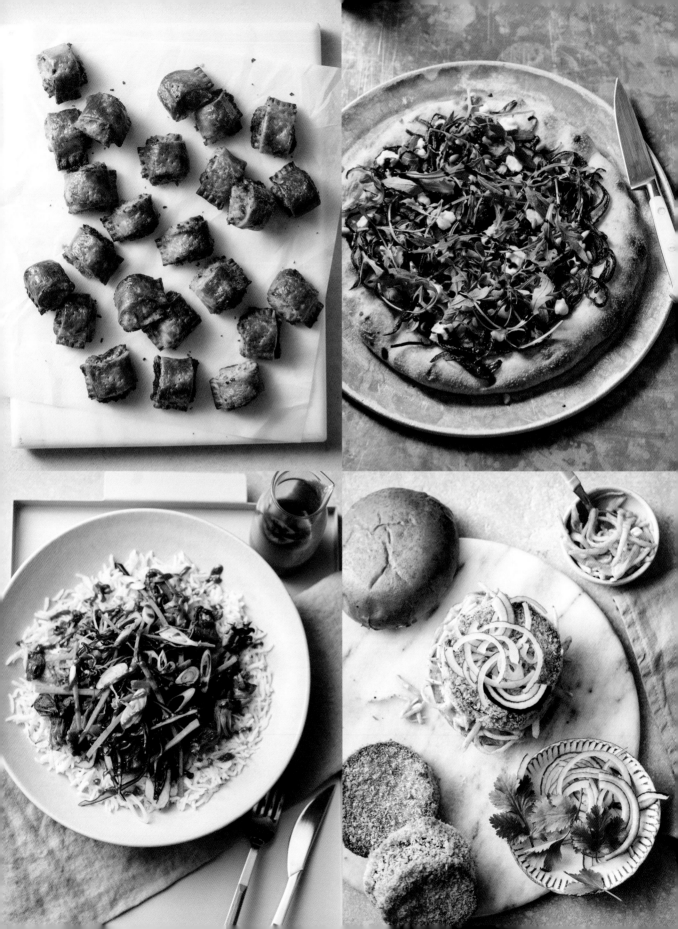

Tandoori Loaded Sweet Potatoes
Nourishing Orzo Soup
Balsamic Red Onion
and Goat's Cheese Pizza
Korean BBQ Jackfruit Rice Bowl
Aubergine Katsu Burger
Roasted Vegetable Paella
Tofu Pad Thai
Cheesy 'Sausage' Rolls
One-pot Greek Orzo
Spicy Cauliflower Steaks
Sticky Aubergine Noodles
Easy Red Lentil Dhal

Tandoori Loaded Sweet Potatoes VE

Everybody loves a baked jacket potato, but have you ever thought of using sweet potatoes instead? I like to top mine with spiced chickpeas cooked in coconut milk with juicy tomatoes. When it's chilly outside, they're a tasty winter warmer.

Per serving:

Carbs: 67.7g

Calories: 415

Fat: 8.1g

Protein: 14.8g

SERVES 2

2 sweet potatoes, cleaned
Low-calorie cooking spray
1 tsp olive oil
1 onion, finely sliced
2 garlic cloves, finely grated
1cm piece of fresh ginger,
    finely grated
2 tsp garam masala
1 tsp chilli powder
1 tsp ground cumin
1 × 400g tin chickpeas, drained
1 × 400g tin chopped tomatoes
100ml light coconut milk
4 spring onions, finely sliced
2 tsp mango chutney
Sea salt
Freshly ground black pepper

1. Preheat the oven to 200°C/180°C Fan/Gas 6.
2. Slice the sweet potatoes three-quarters of the way through at 1cm intervals across. Spray with low calorie-cooking spray, sprinkle with salt and place on a baking tray. Roast for 1 hour, until cooked through.
3. While the sweet potatoes are roasting, heat the olive oil in a non-stick frying pan over a medium heat and fry the onion for 6–8 minutes, until softened and lightly golden.
4. Add the garlic and ginger and fry for a further 2 minutes.
5. Add all the spices and cook for a further minute, stirring well to coat the onion and garlic.
6. Stir through the chickpeas, then the chopped tomatoes and coconut milk. Season well with sea salt and black pepper.
7. Leave to bubble over a low heat, until the sweet potatoes are cooked. You want it to be quite thick, but if it is looking too dry, simply add a splash of water.
8. When the sweet potatoes are ready, remove them from the oven and serve with the chickpea curry over the top, sprinkled with the spring onions and a dollop of mango chutney on each one.

Happier, Healthier, Tastier!

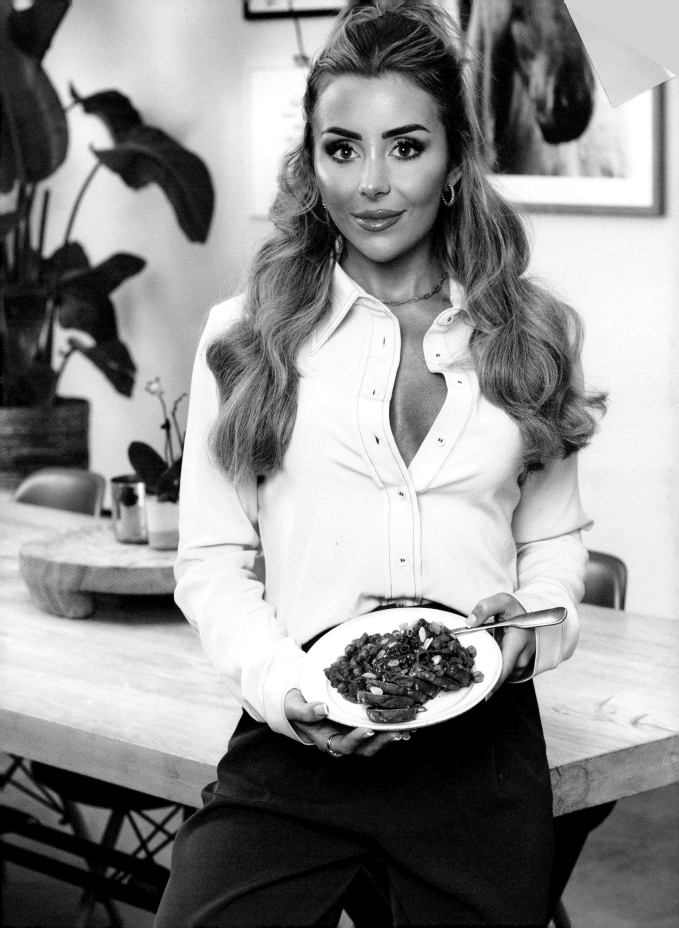

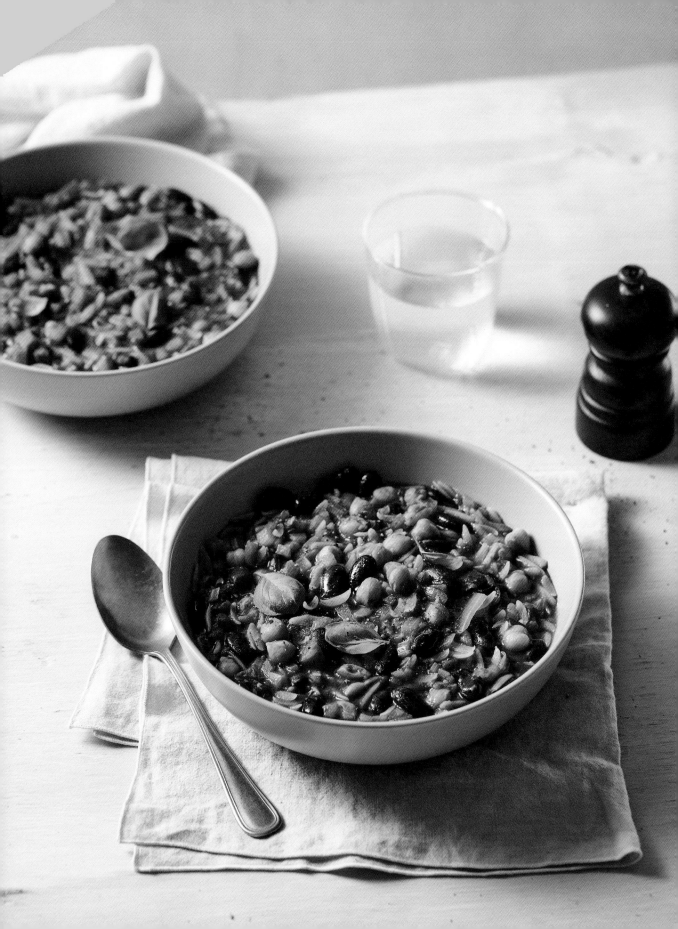

Nourishing Orzo Soup VE

Who could resist this delicious vegan soup on a cold day? It's packed with healthy vegetables, and the beans and chickpeas are a great way to get your daily protein. To make it even more filling, try serving it with a sprinkle of grated reduced-fat vegan cheese. It's a whole meal in a bowl.

Per serving:

Carbs: 45.2g

Calories: 337

Fat: 8.5g

Protein: 10.7g

SERVES 4

2 tbsp olive oil

1 onion, finely diced

2 celery sticks, finely diced

1 carrot, peeled and finely diced

2 garlic cloves, finely grated

1 sprig of rosemary, leaves finely chopped

1 tbsp tomato purée

1 × 400g tin chopped tomatoes

1 × 400g tin red kidney beans, drained

1 × 400g tin chickpeas, drained

150g dried orzo

650ml vegetable stock

½ bunch of fresh basil, finely chopped

Sea salt

Freshly black pepper

1. Heat half the olive oil in a large non-stick saucepan over a medium heat and fry the onion, celery and carrot for 6–8 minutes, until softened.
2. Add the garlic and rosemary, stirring, and cook for 2 minutes.
3. Add the tomato purée and stir well.
4. Add the chopped tomatoes, kidney beans, chickpeas, orzo and vegetable stock and bring to the boil.
5. Reduce the heat and simmer for around 10 minutes, until the orzo is cooked. Season everything well with sea salt and black pepper.
6. Combine the remaining olive oil with the finely chopped basil and drizzle over the top of the soup.

Happier, Healthier, Tastier!

Balsamic Red Onion and Goat's Cheese Pizza Ⓥ

Sweet caramelised red onions and creamy goat's cheese are two of my favourite foods, which is why I adore making these pizzas for an easy supper. With their crispy bases, melted cheese and tangy balsamic glaze, they're irresistible.

Per pizza:

Carbs: 35.8g

Calories: 300

Fat: 14g

Protein: 10g

MAKES 2 PIZZAS

1 tsp olive oil
2 red onions, peeled and very finely sliced
1 tbsp balsamic vinegar
2 tbsp low-fat spread
2 flatbreads
50g soft goat's cheese
2 tbsp pine nuts
2 tbsp balsamic glaze
2 handfuls of rocket leaves
Sea salt
Freshly ground black pepper

1. Preheat the oven to 220°C/200°C Fan/Gas 7.
2. Heat the olive oil over a low heat and add the onions, balsamic vinegar and a couple of tablespoons of water. Cover and cook for 10–15 minutes, until the onions are soft. It may take slightly longer for the liquid to disappear and for the onions to become lightly golden.
3. Spoon the low-fat spread all over the flatbreads, then top with the caramelised onions.
4. Crumble over the goat's cheese and scatter over the pine nuts. Season with sea salt and black pepper.
5. Bake for 15–18 minutes, until the cheese has become gooey and the base is cooked.
6. Serve with the balsamic glaze and a big handful of rocket leaves on each pizza.

Happier, Healthier, Tastier!

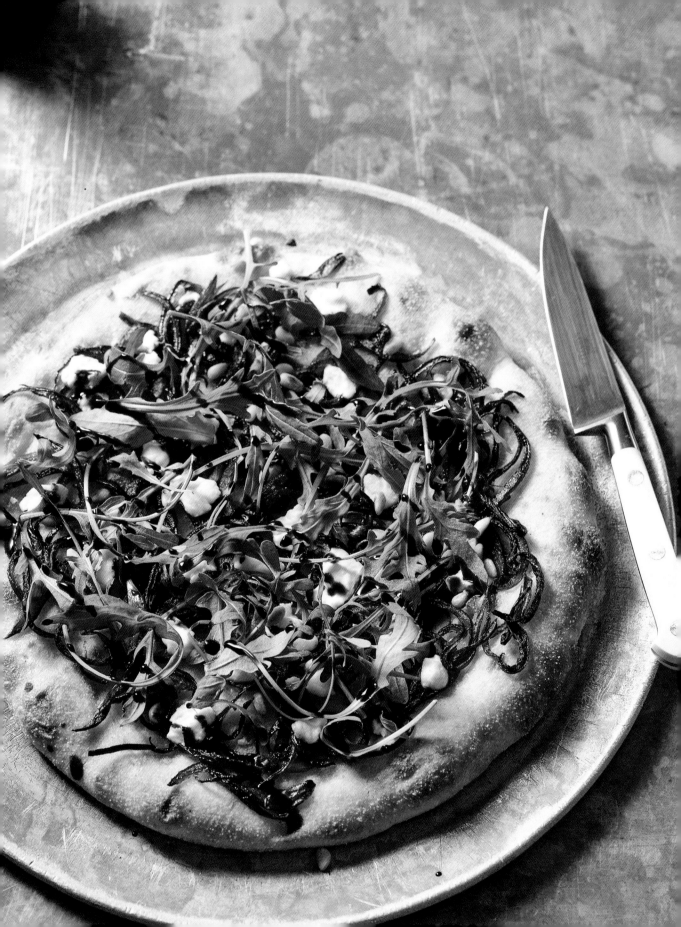

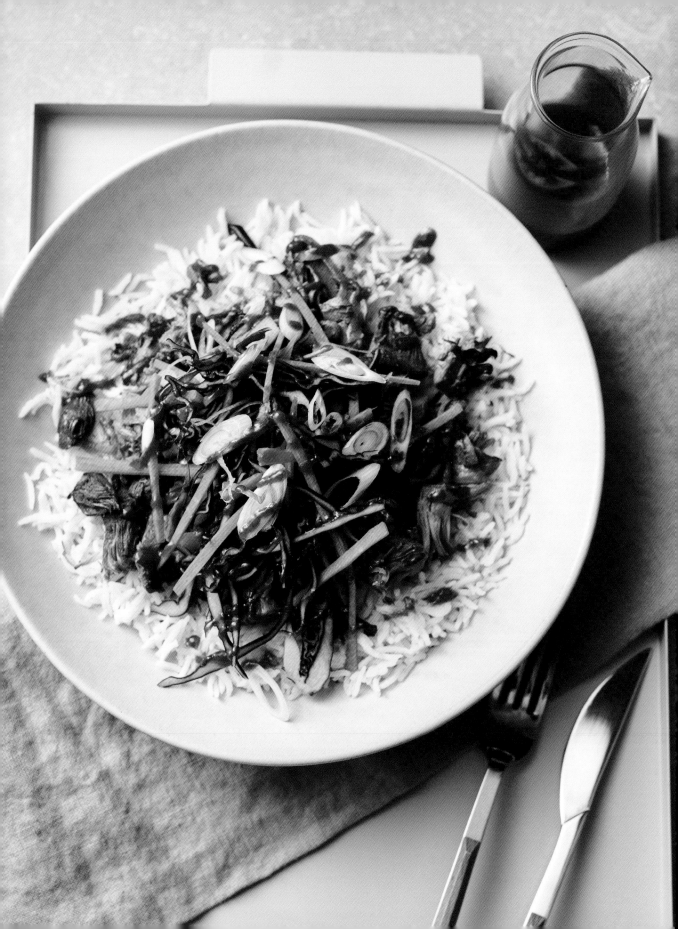

Korean BBQ Jackfruit Rice Bowl VE

Can't believe this is vegan? Well, vegan 'faux meat' substitutes are now really popular, and the best-selling one of all is jackfruit. It's a healthy fruit with a 'meaty' texture, and when you try this delicious little number, you'll be hooked! You need to buy tinned jackfruit in water or brine (not syrup) for this recipe.

Per serving:

Carbs: 84.9g

Calories: 482

Fat: 8.6g

Protein: 11.6g

SERVES 4

1 tbsp olive oil
1 red onion, finely sliced
3 garlic cloves, finely grated
2 tbsp rice vinegar
2 tbsp light soy sauce
1 tbsp sesame oil
2 tbsp Korean-style BBQ sauce
Juice of ½ lime
2 × 410g tins jackfruit, drained and cores removed
300g rice
¼ red cabbage, finely shredded
1 carrot, peeled, halved and cut into thin matchsticks
2 spring onions, finely sliced
Sriracha sauce, for drizzling

1. Heat the olive oil in a large frying pan over a medium heat. Add the sliced onion and cook for 8–10 minutes. Add the garlic and fry for another minute.
2. Meanwhile, mix the rice vinegar, light soy sauce, sesame oil, Korean-style BBQ sauce and lime juice in a small bowl and stir through the jackfruit.
3. Stir the jackfruit and sauce into the pan with the onion and garlic and simmer for 20 minutes, stirring occasionally.
4. Cook the rice according to the packet instructions.
5. Preheat the grill to high, then pop the jackfruit mixture under the grill for 3–5 minutes, until lightly crisp.
6. Divide the rice equally between four bowls, along with a portion of the BBQ jackfruit in each. Top with the cabbage, carrot and spring onions. Drizzle with sriracha sauce.

Happier, Healthier, Tastier!

Aubergine Katsu Burger ⓥ

If you've never been a great aubergine fan, this sweet and spicy plant-based burger will change your mind. Aubergines have become one of the new 'superfood' meat substitutes – and no wonder, when they're so light and healthy and taste so good. And the katsu mayo is so scrummy that you'll soon be serving it with fries, burgers, salads and all your favourite foods.

Per serving:

Carbs: 69.3g

Calories: 320

Fat: 9g

Protein: 10.2g

MAKES 2

40g plain flour
80ml semi-skimmed milk
2 tbsp panko breadcrumbs
1 large aubergine (you'll need 4 thick slices)
Low-calorie cooking spray
3 tbsp light mayonnaise
1 tsp curry powder
1 tsp English mustard
1 tbsp garam masala
2 tsp runny honey
1 tsp soy sauce
¼ white cabbage, very finely shredded
2 brioche burger buns
1 small red onion, very finely sliced
½ bunch of fresh coriander, leaves torn

1. Preheat the oven to 200°C/180°C Fan/Gas 6.
2. In a large bowl, whisk together the plain flour and milk to a smooth batter.
3. Add the panko breadcrumbs to another bowl.
4. Dip the aubergine slices in the batter, then evenly coat with breadcrumbs. Spray well with cooking spray.
5. Place on a wire rack on top of a baking tray and bake in the oven for 25–30 minutes, flipping halfway, until cooked through and golden brown.
6. Meanwhile, combine the mayonnaise, curry powder, English mustard, garam masala, honey and soy sauce in a bowl. This is your katsu mayo. Mix the shredded white cabbage through it.
7. Halve and lightly toast the brioche buns.
8. Divide the aubergine between the bottom halves of the buns, top with the red onion, the katsu slaw and the fresh coriander, then finish with the top halves of the buns.

Happier, Healthier, Tastier!

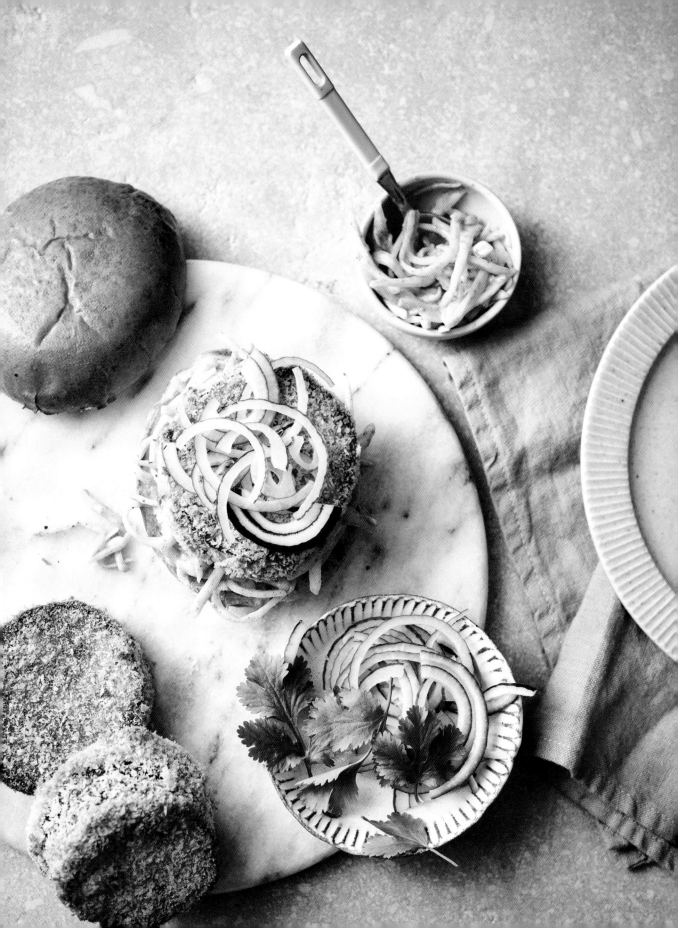

Roasted Vegetable Paella

Per serving:

Carbs: 96.6g

Calories: 523

Fat: 6.6g

Protein: 10.7g

This tasty paella is perfect for lazy days when you don't feel like cooking. After you've prepared the vegetables all you need do is pop them into the oven and, twenty minutes later, add the rice and stock. Wait another twenty minutes and dinner is served. What could be simpler?

SERVES 2

1 courgette, cut into large chunks

1 aubergine, cut into large chunks

1 red pepper, deseeded and cut into large chunks

1 red onion, cut into large chunks

10 cherry tomatoes

Low-calorie cooking spray

200g risotto rice

500ml vegetable stock

2 garlic cloves, finely grated

60g black olives, pitted

Juice of ½ lemon

Sea salt

Freshly ground black pepper

1. Preheat the oven to 200°C/180°C Fan/Gas 6.
2. Place the courgette, aubergine, red pepper, red onion and cherry tomatoes in a deep roasting dish and spray with low-calorie cooking spray. Bake in the oven for 20 minutes.
3. Remove from the oven, add the rice, vegetable stock, garlic and olives to the vegetables and stir through. Return to the oven for a further 20 minutes. Give it a little longer, if needed, until the rice is tender.
4. Squeeze the lemon juice over to serve and season well with sea salt and black pepper.

Happier, Healthier, Tastier!

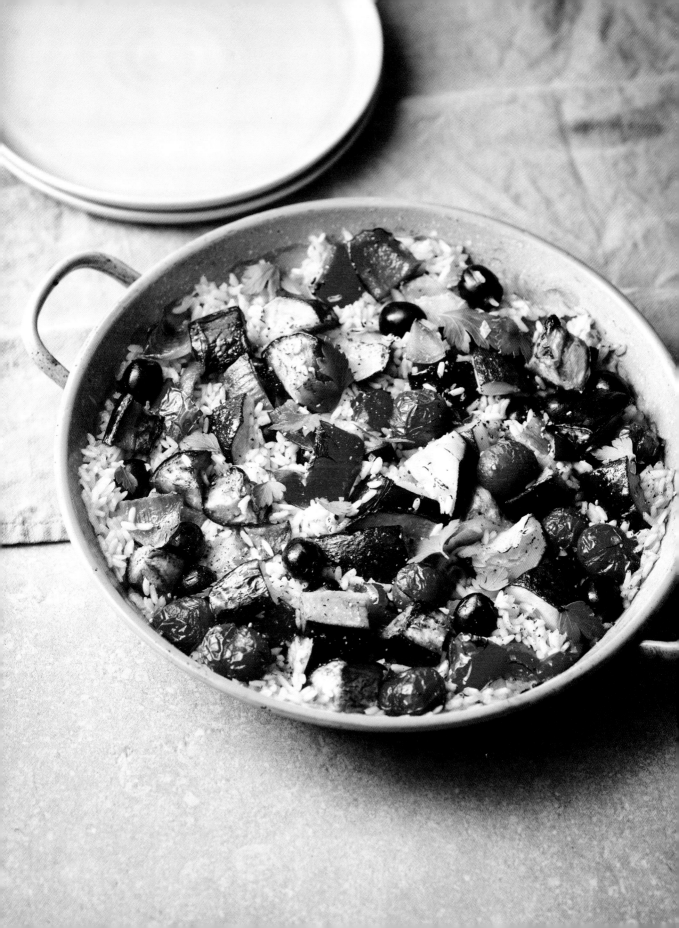

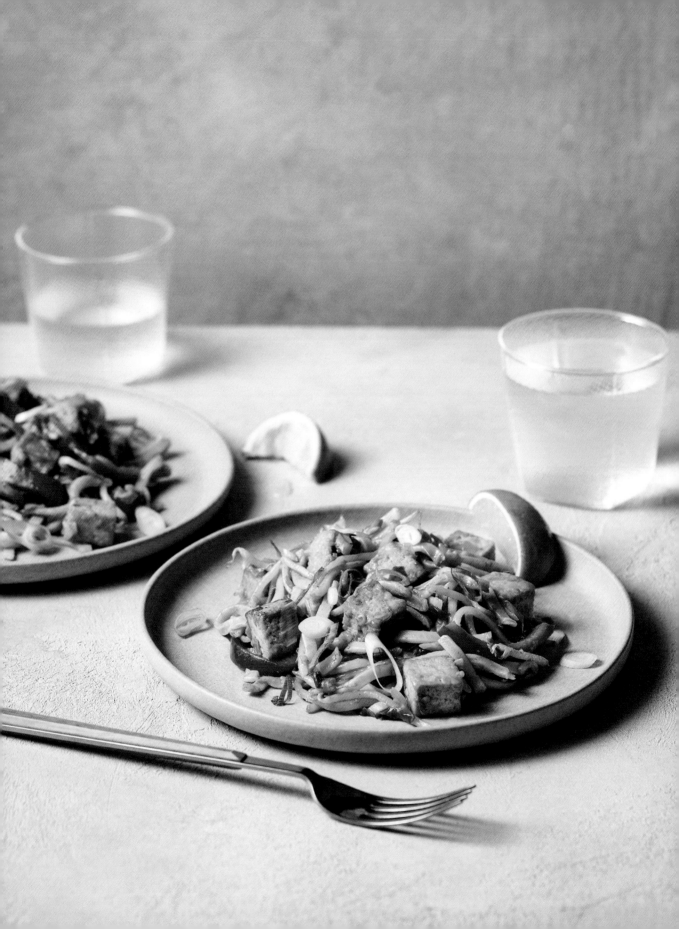

Tofu Pad Thai VE

Per serving:

Carbs: 40g

Calories: 419

Fat: 19.7g

Protein: 24.5g

If you think tofu is boring, this vegan pad Thai will change your mind. Use firm or extra-firm tofu and drain and pat dry with kitchen paper before cooking, until it's appetisingly golden and crispy. Served with rice noodles and vegetables in a wonderful umami sauce, it's the food of the gods.

SERVES 4

1 tbsp maple syrup
1 tbsp tomato ketchup
3 tbsp light soy sauce
Juice of 1 lime
½ tsp cayenne pepper
350g extra-firm tofu, patted dry and cut into cubes
1 heaped tbsp plain flour
2 tbsp olive oil
1 red pepper, deseeded and finely sliced
2 garlic cloves, finely chopped
250g beansprouts
6 spring onions, finely sliced
250g straight-to-wok flat rice noodles
1 lime, cut into wedges

1. Combine the maple syrup, tomato ketchup, soy sauce, lime juice, cayenne pepper and 2 tablespoons water in a small bowl.
2. In another bowl, toss the tofu cubes in the flour to evenly coat.
3. Heat half the oil in a large non-stick frying pan or wok over a medium heat and fry the tofu, until crispy (around 6–8 minutes), then transfer to a plate and set aside.
4. Add the remaining oil to the pan and stir-fry the red pepper over a medium–high heat. Add the garlic, beansprouts and spring onions and fry for a further 2 minutes.
5. Tip the noodles into the pan, along with the cooked tofu and the sauce. Mix everything through for 2 minutes, until the noodles are hot. Serve with lime wedges.

Happier, Healthier, Tastier!

Cheesy 'Sausage' Rolls Ⓥ

If you've never tried veggie sausage rolls, there's no better time than now. They don't take long to assemble, and they cook in fifteen minutes. Eat them as a healthy snack, serve them with pre-dinner drinks or at parties and buffets or enjoy them as a light lunch with a salad. They taste good hot or cold and will reheat well in a hot oven.

Per roll:

Carbs: 9.4g

Calories: 101

Fat: 5.1g

Protein: 4.2g

MAKES 20
Low-calorie cooking spray
1 onion, very finely chopped
2 garlic cloves, finely grated
200g reduced-fat Cheddar, grated
60g panko breadcrumbs
1 tbsp double cream
1 × 375g pack ready-rolled light puff pastry
1 egg, beaten
Freshly ground black pepper

1. Preheat the oven to 220°C/200°C Fan/Gas 7.
2. Spray a medium non-stick frying pan with low-calorie cooking spray over a medium heat and fry the onion for 5–7 minutes, until soft and golden. Add the garlic and fry for a further 2 minutes.
3. Remove from the heat and leave to cool completely.
4. In a large bowl, mix together the cooled onion and garlic, cheese, breadcrumbs and double cream. Season very well with black pepper. Combine everything with your hands really well, until it's all stuck together.
5. Roll out the puff pastry and slice in half lengthways.
6. Spoon the mixture down the middle of each pastry strip right to the ends (but not the sides – leave a little free at the edges).
7. Brush some of the egg along the edge of the pastry, then roll the puff pastry strips over themselves to cover the filling. Use a fork to press where the top and bottom of the pastry connect to hold in place.
8. Slice each one into 10–12 'sausage' rolls, then prick the tops to stop them exploding in the oven.
9. Transfer them to two baking trays and bake in the oven for 15 minutes, until golden and puffed up.

Happier, Healthier, Tastier!

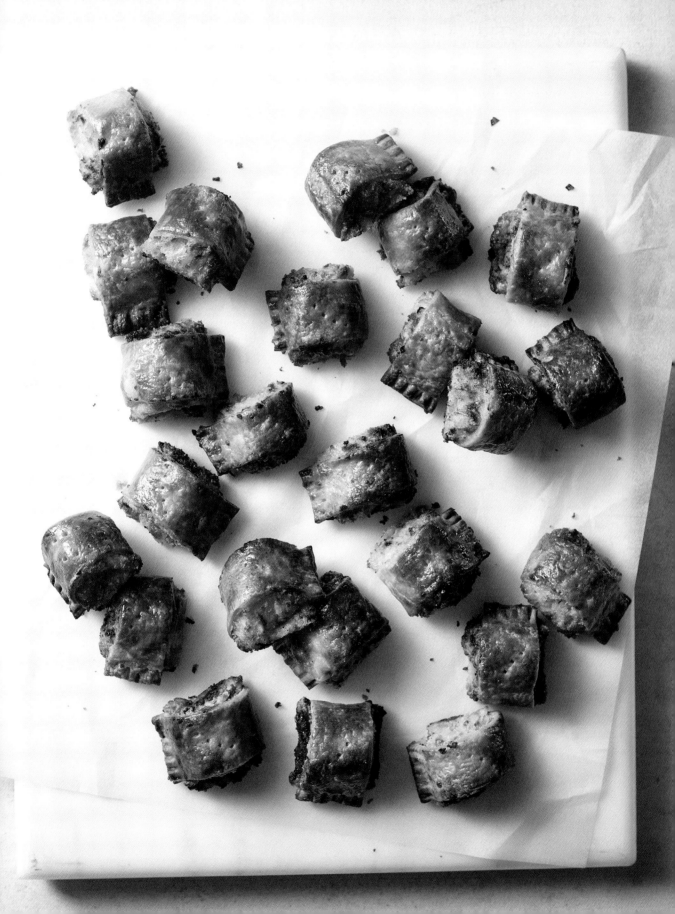

One-pot Greek Orzo ⓥ

Per serving:

Carbs: 37g

Calories: 275

Fat: 8.7g

Protein: 12.2g

What could be more comforting or easy to cook than this? There's virtually no prepping and everything is done in the same pot, so there's minimal washing up and you can just pop the dirty plates and cutlery in the dishwasher, then put your feet up and relax.

SERVES 4

1 tbsp olive oil
1 onion, peeled and finely chopped
1 courgette, trimmed, halved lengthways, then sliced into 1cm pieces
2 garlic cloves, finely grated
1 tsp dried oregano
200g cherry tomatoes
400g orzo
Juice and zest of 1 lemon
800ml vegetable stock
100g reduced-fat feta
Sea salt

1. Heat the olive oil in a large casserole dish over a medium heat and fry the onion and courgette with a sprinkle of sea salt for 4–5 minutes, until softened and lightly golden.
2. Add the garlic and dried oregano and fry for a further 2 minutes.
3. Add the cherry tomatoes and fry for 8–10 minutes, until softened, stirring frequently. You may need to add another splash of oil to the pan if it's a bit dry.
4. Add the orzo and lemon zest and give everything a good stir, then stir through the stock. Simmer over a low–medium heat for 8–10 minutes, until the orzo is cooked and the liquid is more or less absorbed.
5. Squeeze in the lemon juice, then give it a really good stir before crumbling the feta over the top.

Happier, Healthier, Tastier!

Spicy Cauliflower Steaks

Per serving:

Carbs: 36.1g

Calories: 299

Fat: 15.2g

Protein: 9g

Can't believe this is vegan? Well, it turns out that roasted thick slices of cauliflower, dusted with spices, are surprisingly filling and 'meaty'. Plus, they're absolutely delicious, easy to cook and a great low-carb meal – perfect for a midweek pick-me-up.

SERVES 2

250g new potatoes, quartered lengthways

2 tbsp olive oil

½ tsp chilli powder

½ tsp smoked paprika

1 cauliflower, sliced into 2.5cm steaks

150g Tenderstem broccoli, steamed

Sea salt

Freshly ground black pepper

1. Preheat the oven to 220°C/200°C Fan/Gas 7.
2. Place the potato wedges on a baking tray and coat them in 1 tablespoon of the olive oil. Season well with salt and pepper and bake in the oven for around 30 minutes, until crispy and tender.
3. Grab another baking tray and line it with non-stick baking paper.
4. Sprinkle the chilli powder and smoked paprika over the cauliflower steaks and rub them in, followed by the remaining olive oil and rub that in, too.
5. Roast the cauliflower steaks for around 20 minutes, until tender inside and lightly charred.
6. Serve with the steamed broccoli and your favourite sauce.

Happier, Healthier, Tastier!

Sticky Aubergine Noodles (VE)

When you're tired and hungry after a long day at work, it's good to know that you can rustle up these amazing sesame noodles in just fifteen minutes. They're deliciously sweet and spicy and amazingly soothing when you need to just chillax and let all your worries slip away.

Per serving:

Carbs: 67.7g

Calories: 512

Fat: 12.1g

Protein: 8.5g

SERVES 2

1 tbsp sesame oil
2 tbsp maple syrup
1 tbsp light soy sauce
2 garlic cloves, finely grated
1 tbsp finely grated fresh ginger
2 aubergines, trimmed, halved lengthways, then sliced into 2cm pieces
300g straight-to-wok udon noodles
200g green beans, trimmed and each sliced into thirds
4 spring onions, trimmed and finely sliced
1 tbsp sesame seeds

1. Heat a wok or large non-stick frying pan over a medium heat.
2. With a fork, mix together the sesame oil, maple, soy sauce, garlic and ginger in a small bowl.
3. Add the aubergines to the sauce and mix through, until coated.
4. Add to the wok or pan and fry the aubergines for 10 minutes, until soft and cooked through.
5. Add the noodles and green beans and toss to coat in the sauce, until cooked, then serve with the spring onions and sesame seeds on top.

Happier, Healthier, Tastier!

Easy Red Lentil Dhal ⓋⒺ

Per serving:

Carbs: 74.3g

Calories: 551

Fat: 19.2g

Protein: 27.3g

There's always something so comforting about a bowl of steaming, spicy dhal on a cold day. It warms you up, makes you feel full and is a great source of protein, iron and dietary fibre. Adding coconut milk gives the dhal a soothing, creamy texture and wonderful flavour.

SERVES 2

1 tsp coconut oil
1 onion, finely diced
2 tbsp lazy ginger (paste from a jar)
2 tbsp lazy garlic (paste from a jar)
1 tsp ground cumin
1 tsp ground coriander
1 tsp garam masala
2 tsp ground turmeric
1 tsp chilli powder
200g dried red lentils, rinsed
1 × 400g tin light coconut milk
500ml vegetable stock
50g baby spinach
Fresh coriander, leaves torn, to serve
Sea salt
Freshly ground black pepper

1. Heat the coconut oil over a medium heat and fry the onion for 6–7 minutes, until softened and lightly golden.
2. Add the ginger and garlic and fry for a further 2–3 minutes.
3. Sprinkle in all the ground spices and cook for a further minute, stirring well, until the onion is well coated.
4. Add the red lentils and stir them through, then pour in the coconut milk and vegetable stock.
5. Season with salt and pepper and bring to the boil. As soon as it's boiling, reduce the heat and simmer with a lid on for 10 minutes.
6. Remove the lid and simmer for another 10 minutes.
7. Stir through the spinach and cook for a few minutes, until wilted.
8. Serve, sprinkled with the fresh coriander.

Happier, Healthier, Tastier!

Entertaining

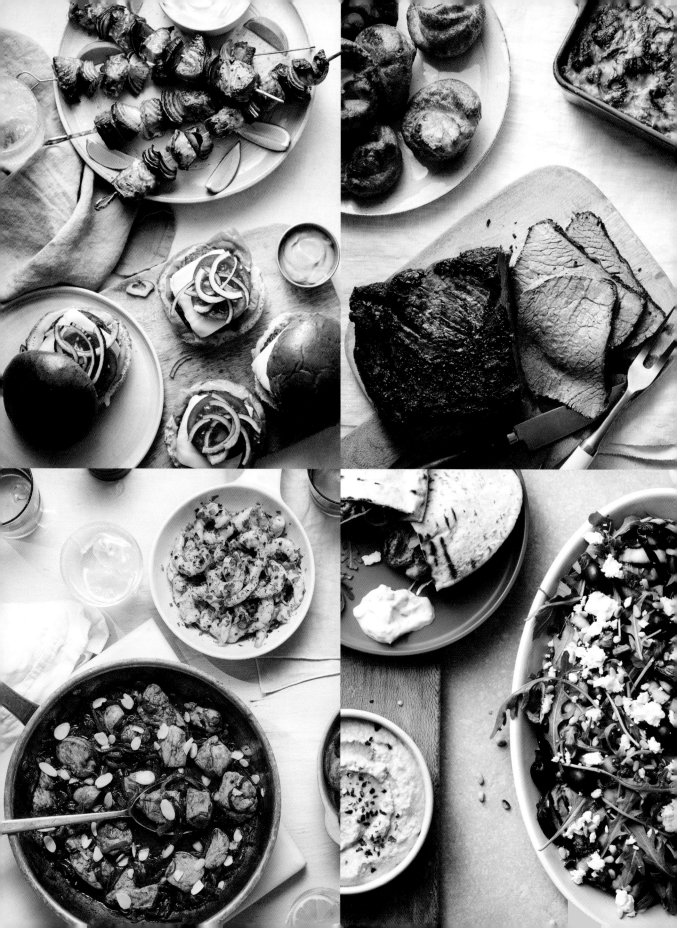

Spanish Fiesta
Whole Roasted Harissa Cauliflower
Turkish Meze
Japanese Restaurant
Chippie Night
Classic Roast Chicken Dinner
Roast Beef with Dauphinoise Potatoes
and Yorkshire Puddings
BBQ Feast
Steak with Chimichurri Sauce

Spanish Fiesta

It's party time and if you're stuck for ideas, we've got you covered. Smash it with our colourful Spanish fiesta menu. It's so easy if you make the Spanish chicken and the chickpea and chorizo salad in advance and reheat them just before serving. That way, you can relax with a pre-dinner glass of wine or dry sherry and get to spend more time with your dinner guests.

Spanish chicken

1 tbsp olive oil
1 red onion, finely sliced
1 red pepper, deseeded and finely sliced
2 boneless, skinless chicken breasts, cut into chunks
½ tsp ground cinnamon
1 tsp smoked paprika
150ml chicken stock
1 tbsp balsamic vinegar
1 tbsp honey
1 tbsp flaked almonds
Sea salt
Freshly ground black pepper

Per serving: Carbs: 8.7g | Calories: 179 | Fat: 7.3g | Protein: 15.9g

1. Heat the olive oil in a medium non-stick pan and fry the onion and pepper for 5 minutes, until softened.
2. Add the chicken to the pan and fry, until golden brown.
3. Stir through the cinnamon and smoked paprika and fry for around 1 minute.
4. Pour in the chicken stock, balsamic vinegar and honey and bring to the boil. Season with sea salt and black pepper.
5. Immediately reduce the heat and simmer for 15 minutes, until the sauce has thickened and the chicken is cooked through.
6. Serve with the flaked almonds scattered over the top.

Garlic chilli prawns

1 tbsp olive oil
1 tsp dried chilli flakes
4 garlic cloves, finely chopped
Juice of ½ lemon
20 raw king prawns
1 tbsp flat-leaf parsley, finely chopped
Freshly ground black pepper

Per serving: Carbs: 1g | Calories: 70 | Fat: 3.7g | Protein: 8.4g

1. Heat the olive oil in a large non-stick frying pan over a low–medium heat. Add the chilli flakes and garlic. It is really important that your pan is not too hot, otherwise the garlic will burn very quickly. Keep an eye on the garlic and if it begins to brown, remove from the heat.
2. Once the garlic smells fragrant, increase the heat and add the lemon juice to stop the frying process.
3. Add the prawns to the pan and fry for 1 minute on each side. The prawns are cooked when they are pink – don't overcook them.
4. Season with black pepper and scatter over the parsley to serve.

Happier, Healthier, Tastier!

Patatas bravas (v)

800g new potatoes, halved
2 tbsp olive oil
1 onion, finely chopped
2 garlic cloves, finely chopped
1 tsp smoked paprika
1 × 400g tin chopped tomatoes
1 tsp honey
Sea salt
Freshly ground black pepper

Per serving: Carbs: 37.8g | Calories: 236 | Fat: 7.2g | Protein: 4g

1. Boil the potatoes in salted water for 10–12 minutes in a medium saucepan over a high heat, until nearly cooked through. Drain and leave to steam-dry while you make the sauce.
2. Heat half the olive oil in a large-non-stick frying pan and fry the onion for 4 minutes, until softened.
3. Add the garlic and fry for a further minute, then sprinkle in the smoked paprika and fry for another minute.
4. Add the chopped tomatoes and honey and season well with sea salt and black pepper. Simmer over a low heat for 10–15 minutes, until thickened.
5. Grab another frying pan and place over a high heat. Add the remaining olive oil and fry the potatoes for around 10 minutes, until lightly crisp.
6. Transfer the potatoes to a large bowl and spoon over the delicious smoky tomato sauce.

Chickpea and chorizo salad

225g reduced-fat chorizo ring, sliced
1 × 480g jar roasted red peppers, drained and finely sliced
1 × 400g tin chickpeas, drained
½ bunch fresh coriander, roughly chopped
80g rocket leaves
4 tbsp fat-free yoghurt
Freshly ground black pepper

Per serving: Carbs: 6.2g | Calories: 230 | Fat: 14.7g | Protein: 17.4g

1. Heat a large non-stick frying pan over a medium heat and fry the chorizo for 10 minutes, until golden and lightly crisp. The chorizo will release its own oil as it cooks.
2. Stir in the roasted red peppers and chickpeas and warm through.
3. Transfer to a large plate or bowl, scatter over the coriander and rocket leaves, then spoon over the yoghurt and season with black pepper.

Happier, Healthier, Tastier!

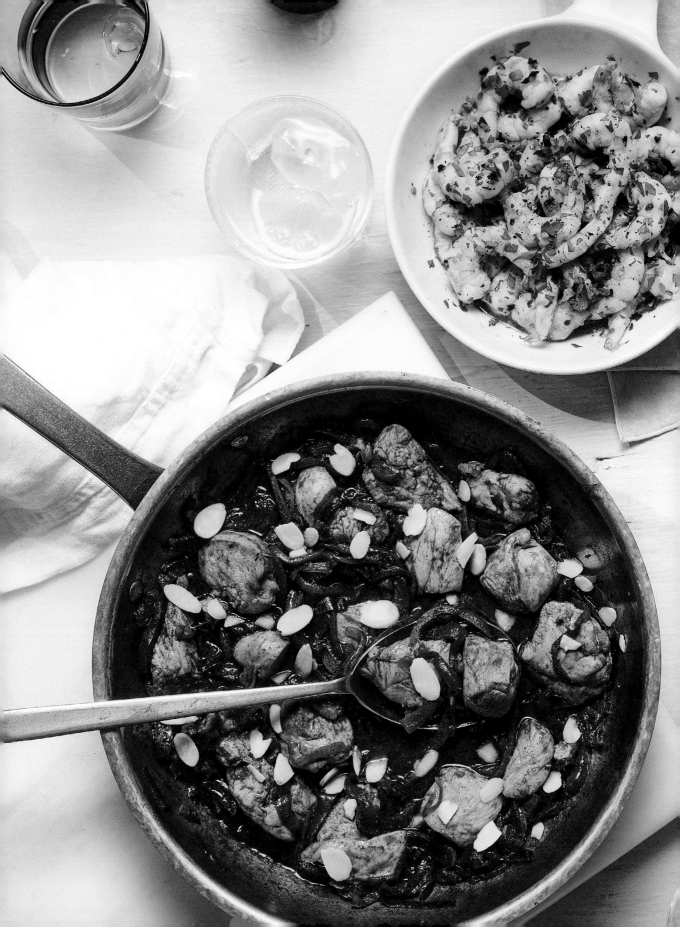

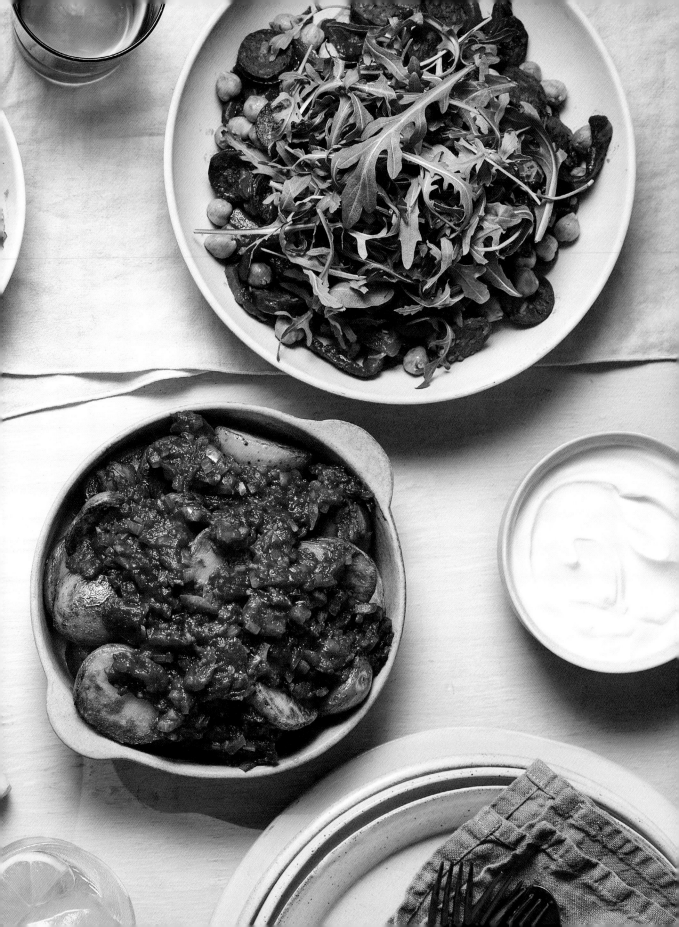

Whole Roasted Harissa Cauliflower

SERVES 4

A whole roasted cauliflower looks so impressive and will easily be the centrepiece of your table. And what's even better is that it takes only a few minutes to prepare. You can pop it in the oven and get on with preparing the couscous salad and vegetable sides of charred broccoli and maple-glazed carrots while it cooks. It's the perfect feast for when you're entertaining vegan or vegetarian guests.

Roasted harissa cauliflower

1 tsp ground cumin
1 tsp ground turmeric
1 tsp ground paprika
½ tsp ground cinnamon
2 tbsp rose harissa paste
1 tbsp olive oil
1 large head cauliflower, leaves removed
2 tbsp flaked almonds
4 tbsp pomegranate seeds
¼ bunch of fresh coriander, leaves torn
Sea salt
Freshly ground black pepper

Per serving: Carbs: 14.6g | Calories: 149 | Fat: 6.2g | Protein: 6.1g

1. Preheat the oven to 200°C/180°C Fan/Gas 6.
2. In a large bowl, combine all the ground spices with half the harissa paste and the olive oil. Add a good pinch of sea salt and black pepper.
3. Add the cauliflower to the bowl and stir everything well, rubbing the spice mix well into the cauliflower.
4. Pop the cauliflower on a lined baking tray and bake in the oven for around 1½ hours, until tender.
5. Remove from the oven and scatter over the flaked almonds, pomegranate seeds and fresh coriander.

Couscous salad

300g couscous
450ml vegetable stock
10g flat-leaf parsley, chopped
10g fresh coriander, chopped
Juice and zest of 1 lemon
1 tbsp olive oil
2 tbsp raisins
50g vegan feta, crumbled
Freshly ground black pepper

Per serving: Carbs: 32g | Calories: 219 | Fat: 7.2g | Protein: 5.5g

1. Cook the couscous in the vegetable stock, according to the packet instructions, with a pinch of black pepper.
2. Fluff with a fork and stir through the parsley, coriander, lemon juice and zest, olive oil and raisins and crumble over the vegan feta.

Happier, Healthier, Tastier!

Broccoli with tahini dressing

600g Tenderstem broccoli
2 tbsp tahini
1 tsp olive oil
Juice of ½ lemon
1 tsp maple syrup
1 tsp sesame seeds

Per serving: Carbs: 7.4g | Calories: 119 | Fat: 5.8g | Protein: 7.3g

1. In a medium saucepan, cook the broccoli for 2–3 minutes in boiling water over a high heat.
2. While the broccoli is cooking, mix the tahini, olive oil, lemon juice and maple syrup in a small bowl.
3. Toast the sesame seeds in a small pan over a high heat, tossing until lightly golden.
4. Drain the broccoli and, while it's still warm, pour over the tahini sauce and scatter with the toasted sesame seeds.

Maple-glazed carrots

300g carrots, quartered lengthways, so they're long strips
2 tbsp maple syrup
1 tbsp wholegrain mustard
1 tbsp olive oil
Sea salt
Freshly ground black pepper

Per serving: Carbs: 14.2g | Calories: 88 | Fat: 3.6g | Protein: 0.7g

1. Preheat the oven to 200°C/180°C Fan/Gas 6.
2. Place the carrots in a medium saucepan of boiling water and cook for 5 minutes over a high heat. Drain and transfer to a roasting tray and arrange in a single layer.
3. Mix the maple syrup, mustard and olive oil through the carrots, sprinkle with salt and pepper and roast for 30–35 minutes, until tender and golden.

Happier, Healthier, Tastier!

Turkish Meze

SERVES 8

Sharing is caring, and what could be a better way of doing that than with a traditional table of delicious meze sharing plates. This is effortless entertaining at its best! Prepare the kofta mixture, salad and dips ahead of time, and it's in the bag. Then the only things left to do are to lay the table and grill the skewered koftas just before you sit down to eat.

Lamb koftas

500g lean lamb mince
1 tsp ground coriander
2 tsp ground cumin
2 garlic cloves, finely grated
Low-calorie cooking spray
8 pitta breads

Per serving: Carbs: 28g | Calories: 280 | Fat: 10.6g | Protein: 16.5g

1. In a large bowl, combine the lamb mince, ground coriander, ground cumin and garlic with your hands for a couple of minutes. The longer you combine it for, the better the koftas will hold together.
2. Divide the mixture into balls, then push on to metal skewers (allow two per skewer) and spray all over with cooking spray.
3. Heat a large non-stick frying pan or griddle pan over a medium–high heat, then place the koftas in the pan, only turning once they have turned a deep golden brown on that side. It should take around 4 minutes per side.
4. Turn the grill to high, place the pitta breads on a baking tray and grill for around 30 seconds on each side, until puffed up and golden.
5. Slice the pitta breads open and serve with the lamb koftas inside. You can also load the pitta breads with the sides below and opposite.

Tzatziki

500g fat-free yoghurt
½ garlic clove, finely grated
1 large cucumber, halved lengthways, deseeded and grated
2 spring onions, finely chopped
Small handful of fresh mint, finely chopped
Sea salt
Freshly ground black pepper

Per serving: Carbs: 2.4g | Calories: 24 | Fat: 0.1g | Protein: 2.4g

1. Combine the yoghurt, garlic, cucumber, spring onions and mint in a small bowl.
2. Season with sea salt and black pepper and mix well.

Happier, Healthier, Tastier!

Grilled aubergine salad Ⓞ

2 tbsp pine nuts
3 aubergines, ends cut off
  and sliced lengthways into
  pieces 1cm thick
Low-calorie cooking spray
2 tbsp olive oil
1 tbsp balsamic vinegar
½ garlic clove, finely grated
1 small bunch of fresh
  coriander, roughly chopped
60g rocket leaves (or your
  preferred salad leaves)
Handful of black olives, pitted
150g reduced-fat feta,
  crumbled
Sea salt

Per serving: Carbs: 1.3g | Calories: 100 | Fat: 5.9g | Protein: 3.8g

1. Toast the pine nuts in a dry frying pan until lightly golden. Remove from the pan and set aside.
2. Place the aubergine slices in a bowl, season with sea salt, then spray well with low-calorie cooking spray and toss to combine.
3. Heat a griddle pan over a medium–high heat and grill the aubergines in batches, not moving them too much to ensure nice char marks. They should take around 3 minutes on each side.
4. Make a dressing by combining the olive oil, balsamic vinegar, garlic and the fresh coriander.
5. Mix the dressing through the salad leaves, then add to a large bowl. Lay the grilled aubergine slices in and around the salad, then sprinkle over the olives and crumbled feta. Finish by sprinkling over the toasted pine nuts.

Hummus Ⓞ

2 × 400g tins chickpeas (liquid
  reserved)
4 tsp tahini
½ tsp ground cumin
1 garlic clove
Juice of ½ lemon
Sea salt
Freshly ground black pepper
½ tsp dried chilli flakes, to
  serve
1 tsp cumin seeds, to serve

Per serving: Carbs: 10.6g | Calories: 119 | Fat: 5.6g | Protein: 5.1g

1. Add the chickpeas, the tahini, cumin, garlic and lemon juice to a food processor.
2. Turn the processor on and slowly add some of the reserved chickpea liquid, a tablespoon at a time, until you begin to get a smooth mixture. You'll need around 5 tablespoons in total.
3. With the blade still running, add the olive oil to create a silky hummus.
4. Spoon the hummus into a serving dish and top with a sprinkle of the dried chilli flakes and cumin seeds.

Happier, Healthier, Tastier!

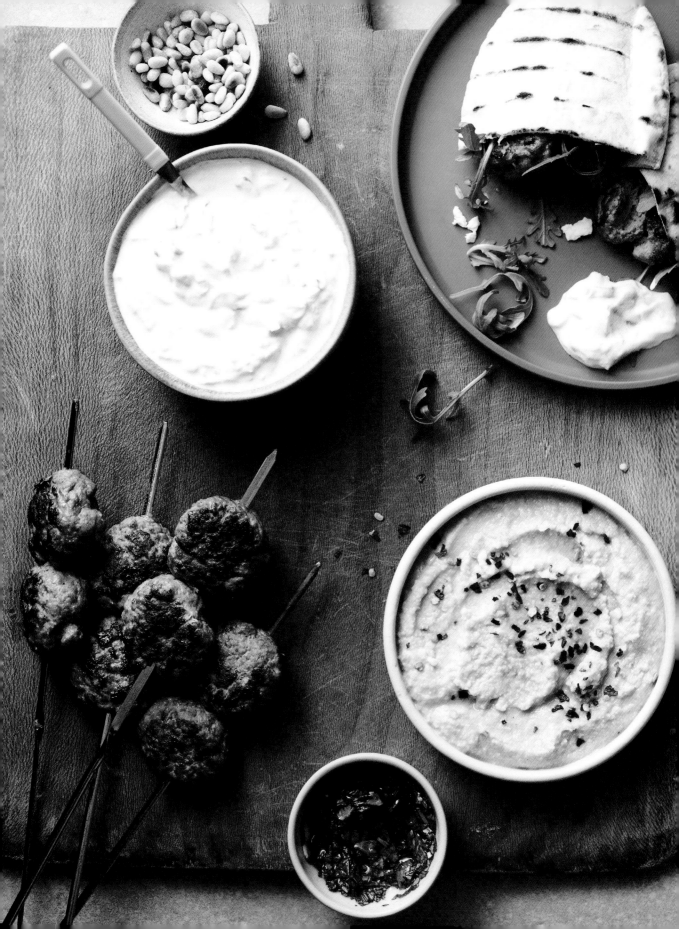

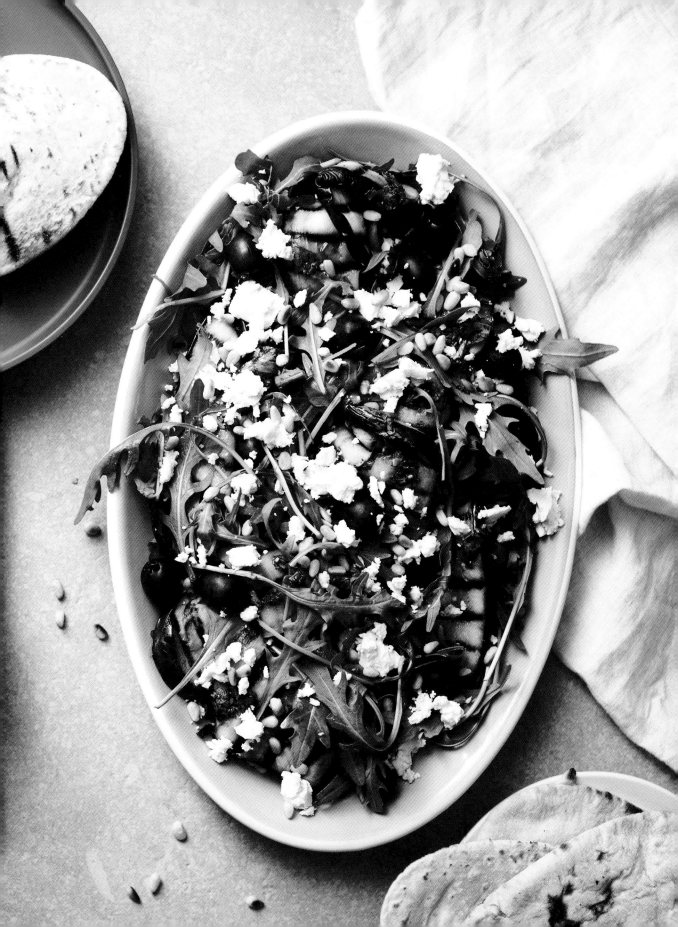

Japanese Restaurant

Japanese food, with its distinctive umami flavours, has taken the world by storm, but you don't have to go to a restaurant or order a takeaway to enjoy it. Try cooking this easy Japanese feast at home – all the dishes are simple to make and the ingredients are all available in your local supermarket. So get shopping and cooking.

Chicken katsu

1 large egg, beaten
10 tbsp cornflakes, finely crushed with your hands
4 skinless, boneless chicken breasts
1 garlic clove, finely grated
2 tbsp korma paste
1 tbsp dark soy sauce
3 tbsp ketchup
2 tbsp honey
2 tbsp cornflour
2 × 250g pouches ready-cooked microwave jasmine rice
1 red onion, finely sliced
½ bunch of fresh coriander, leaves torn
1 tsp black sesame seeds (optional)

Per serving: Calories: | Carbs: 54.9g 446 | Fat: 7g | Protein: 41.1g

1. Preheat the oven to 200°C/180°C Fan/Gas 6 and line a small baking tray with non-stick baking paper.
2. Take two plates and add the beaten egg to one and the cornflakes to the other.
3. Dip the chicken breasts in the egg, then coat entirely in cornflakes.
4. Place the chicken on the prepared baking tray and bake in the oven for around 20–25 minutes, until cooked through completely – when no pink remains and the juices run clear.
5. Place the garlic, korma paste, soy sauce, ketchup, honey and cornflour in a large non-stick saucepan over a medium heat, then pour in 450ml water. Whisk together, until smooth, then bring to the boil gradually, still on medium heat, until the cornflour has thickened the sauce. Cover the pan, so it doesn't thicken further, then cook over a low heat for around 5 minutes.
6. Microwave the rice according to the packet instructions, then divide between four bowls.
7. Slice the chicken and place on the rice, then spoon over the delicious katsu sauce and finish by sprinkling over the red onion, fresh coriander and sesame seeds, if using.

Happier, Healthier, Tastier!

Edamame salad (v)

200g Tenderstem broccoli, trimmed and halved
1 tbsp dark soy sauce
1 tsp toasted sesame oil
1 red chilli, deseeded and finely sliced
1 tsp honey
300g edamame beans

Per serving: Carbs: 10.8g | Calories: 118 | Fat: 5.1g | Protein: 9.7g

1. Add the broccoli to a pan of boiling water and cook for 3 minutes, until cooked but still crunchy.
2. Whisk together the soy sauce, sesame oil, red chilli and honey in a small bowl.
3. Drain the broccoli and transfer to a bowl with the edamame beans. Mix through the sesame sauce and serve.

Teriyaki pork lettuce cups

1 tsp olive oil
Thumb-sized piece of fresh ginger, finely grated
2 garlic cloves, finely grated
400g lean pork mince
1 tbsp dark soy sauce
3 tbsp teriyaki sauce
16 Little Gem lettuce leaves
1 red chilli, deseeded and sliced into fine strips

Per serving: Carbs: 4.5g | Calories: 181 | Fat: 6.9g | Protein: 25.2g

1. Heat the olive oil in a frying pan over a medium–high heat and fry the ginger and garlic for 1 minute, stirring constantly so they don't burn.
2. Add the pork mince to the pan, breaking it up with a wooden spoon. Fry for around 8 minutes, until golden brown.
3. Add the soy sauce and teriyaki sauce and stir well to coat the mince. Reduce the heat slightly and let it bubble for a couple of minutes. Load into the lettuce 'cups' and top with the red chilli.

Happier, Healthier, Tastier!

Chippie Night

Who said fish and chips are unhealthy? They're certainly not when you bake succulent cod fillets in my delish crispy coating and serve them with oven-cooked chips, low-cal curry sauce and creamy mushy peas. You'll end up with under half the fat and calories you'd get in the usual chippie takeaway – and it tastes absolutely fabulous.

Chip-shop chips

3 large potatoes, peeled and cut into chips
1 tbsp olive oil
Sea salt

Per serving: Carbs: 47.3g | Calories: 238 | Fat: 3.7g | Protein: 5.3g

1. Preheat the oven to 220°C/200°C Fan/Gas 7. Line a baking tray with non-stick baking paper.
2. Cook the potatoes in a pan of boiling water for 3–4 minutes over a high heat, then drain and leave to steam-dry slightly.
3. Spread the potatoes on the lined baking tray, drizzle with the olive oil and season very generously with sea salt.
4. Bake in the oven for 20–30 minutes, until cooked through, golden and crisp.

Battered cod

2 tbsp plain flour
2 large eggs, beaten
120g cornflakes, bashed in a bag with a rolling pin, until crushed
4 cod fillets
Low-calorie cooking spray
Sea salt
Freshly ground black pepper

Per serving: Carbs: 27.2g | Calories: 265 | Fat: 3.7g | Protein: 30.6g

1. Preheat the oven to 220°C/200°C Fan/Gas 7. Line a large baking tray with non-stick baking paper.
2. Grab three plates: add the plain flour to the first and season it well with sea salt and black pepper; add the beaten eggs to the second; and add the cornflakes to the third, .
3. Dust the fish in the flour, then dredge in the beaten egg and coat evenly in the cornflake crumbs.
4. Pop the fish on the prepared baking tray, spray with low-calorie cooking spray and bake for 20 minutes, until cooked through.

Happier, Healthier, Tastier!

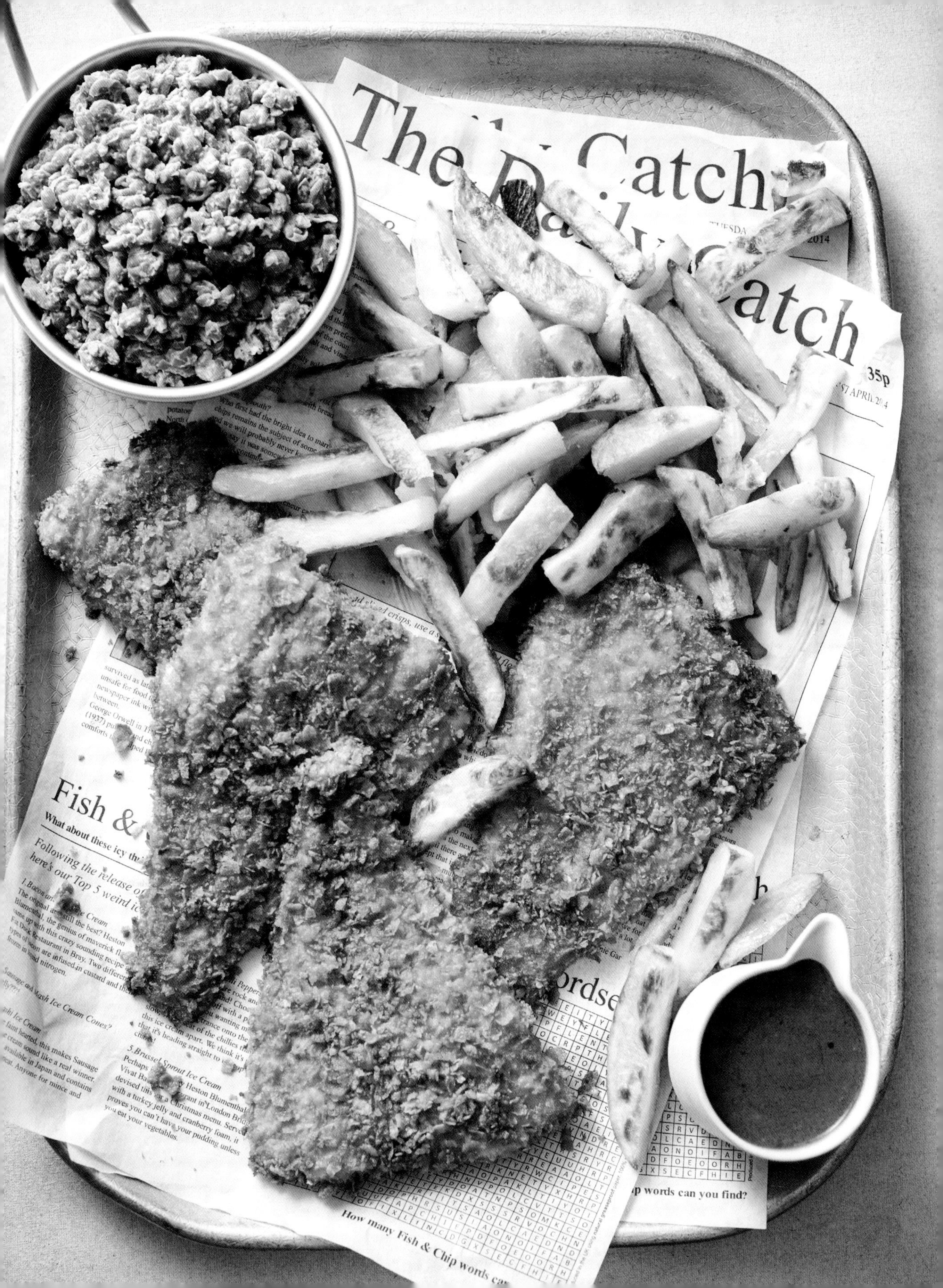

atch
35p
Fish &
What about these icy
Following the release
here's our Top 5 weird
George Orwell
Sausage and Mash Ice Cream Cones?
5.Brussel Sprout Ice Cream
with a turkey jelly and cranberry foam, it
proves you can't have your pudding unless
you eat your vegetables.
words can you find?
How many Fish & Chip words

Curry sauce

350ml chicken stock
1 tbsp curry powder
1 tsp Chinese five-spice
   powder
½ tsp ground turmeric
1 tsp cornflour
1 tbsp plain flour
1 tsp honey
½ tsp paprika
½ tsp salt

Per serving: Carbs: 3.6g | Calories: 41 | Fat: 2.6g | Protein: 3.5g

1. Place all the ingredients in a medium non-stick saucepan over a medium–low heat, whisking constantly, until thickened.

Mushy peas (v)

500g frozen peas
50g low-fat spread
2 tbsp malt vinegar
1 tbsp reduced-fat crème
   fraîche
Sea salt
Freshly ground black pepper

Per serving: Carbs: 16.1g | Calories: 161 | Fat: 6.8g | Protein: 7g

1. Cook the peas in boiling water over a high heat for up to 10 minutes, until soft.
2. Drain and mash very well with the low-fat spread, vinegar, sea salt and black pepper, then stir through the crème fraîche.

Happier, Healthier, Tastier!

Classic Roast Chicken Dinner

SERVES 6

Nothing beats a Sunday roast with family and friends – everybody loves it. The secret to success is all in the timing, which I've perfected over the years. You can rest your roast chicken for up to an hour while you finish cooking the vegetables and make the gravy. This meal doesn't include green vegetables, but boil whichever you prefer and serve them alongside.

Roast chicken

1 garlic bulb, unpeeled and sliced in half horizontally
3 onions, unpeeled and quartered through the root, so they stay intact
2 leeks, trimmed and halved lengthways, then again horizontally
2 large carrots, unpeeled and sliced into thirds
2 sprigs of fresh rosemary
1 chicken stock pot
1.8kg chicken
Low-calorie cooking spray
1 lemon
Sea salt
Freshly ground black pepper

Per serving: Carbs: 4g | Calories: 275 | Fat: 15.7g | Protein: 36.9g

1. Preheat the oven to 200°C/180°C Fan/Gas 6.
2. Place the halved garlic bulb, onions, leeks, carrots, rosemary and chicken stock pot in a large roasting tray with a splash of water.
3. Pop the chicken on top, spray well with low-calorie cooking spray and season generously with sea salt and black pepper. Tuck the lemon inside the chicken cavity.
4. Bake in the oven for around 1 hour 50 minutes or as stated on the chicken packaging. When it's cooked, the juices should run clear when pierced with a sharp knife at the thickest part.
5. Remove from the oven, transfer to a plate, cover with foil and set aside for 30–60 minutes to rest. This ensures juicy meat. Don't worry: your chicken will stay hot for up to 1 hour.

Cauliflower cheese Ⓥ

1 large cauliflower head, cut into large florets, leaves too
85g low-fat spread
85g plain flour
1 litre semi-skimmed milk
100g reduced-fat Cheddar, grated
Sea salt
Freshly ground black pepper

Per serving: Carbs: 24.6g | Calories: 264 | Fat: 11.9g | Protein: 13.6g

1. Cook the cauliflower florets in a medium saucepan of salted boiling water over a high heat for 3 minutes, until tender, then drain in a colander.
2. In another saucepan, melt the spread over a low–medium heat and, once melted, whisk in the flour until you have a thick paste. Slowly add the milk, whisking until it has been absorbed before adding more. Keep going, whisking constantly, until you've used all the milk and the sauce is thick. Season generously with black pepper.
3. Stir in the cheese, until melted, then add the cauliflower and mix through well.
4. Transfer to a large casserole dish and bake in the oven for around 18–20 minutes, until it is bubbling and golden.

Happier, Healthier, Tastier!

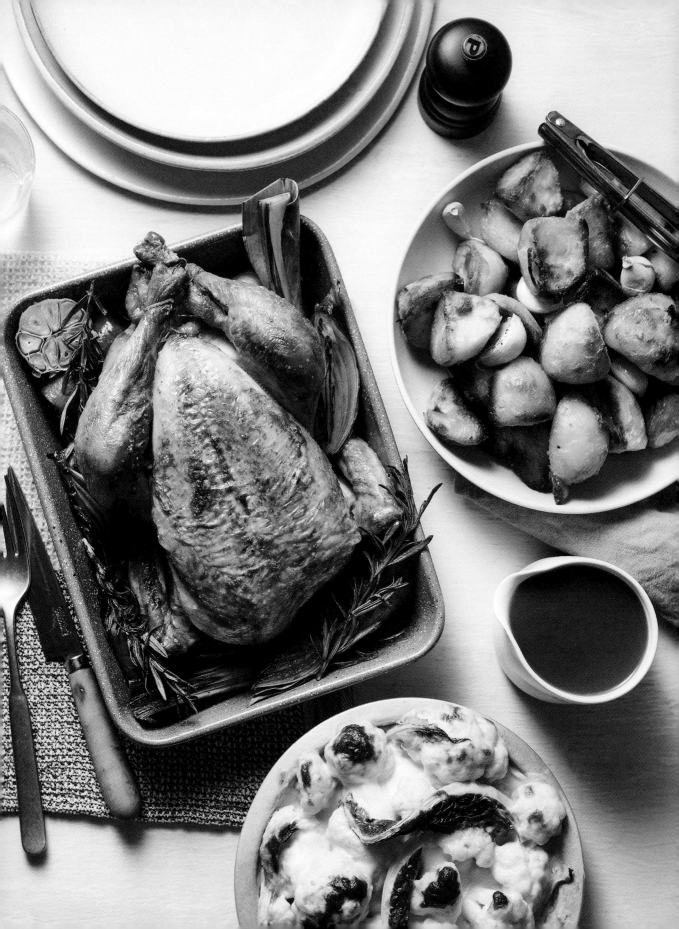

Gravy

Juices from the roasting tray
(see page 189)
2 tbsp plain flour
½ litre chicken stock
Splash of balsamic vinegar
(optional)
Squeeze of honey (optional)

Per serving: Carbs: 2g | Calories: 56 | Fat: 0g | Protein: 0.3g

1. When the chicken has finished cooking, check that your roasting tray can go on the hob, place it over a medium heat, then sprinkle the flour over the vegetables and juices, stirring well and scraping all the bits off the bottom of the tray.
2. When the white flour has disappeared into the sauce/vegetables, pour in the chicken stock and bring to the boil.
3. If the chicken has released any more juices on to the plate it's resting on, add those to the roasting tin, too.
4. Reduce the heat to a simmer and leave to bubble gently for around 4–5 minutes, until thickened. Add a splash of balsamic vinegar and a squeeze of honey (if using).
5. You can either strain for a smooth gravy or keep it rustic with the vegetables still in it.

Garlic roast potatoes Ⓥ

1.2kg potatoes (such as Maris
Piper), peeled and quartered
1 heaped tbsp plain flour
4 tbsp olive oil
6 garlic cloves
Sea salt
Freshly ground black pepper

Per serving: Carbs: 37g | Calories: 251 | Fat: 10g | Protein: 3.9g

1. Preheat the oven to 200°C/180°C Fan/Gas 6.
2. Parboil your potatoes in salted boiling water in a medium saucepan over a high heat for 5 minutes, then drain and leave to steam-dry for 1–2 minutes.
3. Toss the potatoes in the flour to rough up the edges.
4. Pour the olive oil into a large roasting tray and place in the oven for 2 minutes to heat it.
5. Remove the tray from the oven and carefully add the potatoes, spooning the hot oil over them to ensure they are well coated.
6. Scatter over the garlic cloves, then place the tray in the oven and roast the potatoes for 50–60 minutes, until golden and crisp. You may find that flipping them a couple of times during cooking helps to evenly crisp them.
7. Season with a good amount of sea salt and black pepper before serving. Don't forget to squeeze the roasted garlic cloves out of their skins and enjoy!

Happier, Healthier, Tastier!

Roast Beef with Dauphinoise Potatoes and Yorkshire Puddings

SERVES 6

This has got to be the best Sunday roast lunch ever! Tender roast beef served with a creamy, cheesy potato bake and crispy golden Yorkshires. You may need to adjust the cooking times, depending on how rare or well cooked you like your beef. Use a really lean cut, like rolled sirloin, rib of beef or topside.

Roast beef

2kg beef roasting joint
1 tbsp Dijon mustard
1 tbsp plain flour
400ml beef stock
Sea salt
Freshly ground black pepper

Per serving: Carbs: 14.2g | Calories: 581 | Fat: 33.7g | Protein: 68.5g

1. Preheat the oven to 220°C/200°C Fan/Gas 7 and remove the beef from the fridge 30 minutes before cooking.
2. Rub the beef all over with the Dijon mustard and then season well with sea salt and black pepper. Place in a roasting tray.
3. To cook the beef, it takes around 18 minutes per 500g, so check the meat's packaging to determine the weight, then add on a further 20 minutes on top of that. It helps if you tie your beef with kitchen string at regular intervals, but it's not essential.
4. After the beef has been roasting for 35 minutes, reduce the heat to 180°C/160°C Fan/Gas 4 for the remainder of the cooking time. Make sure you spoon over the juices from the bottom of the roasting tray as it cooks to help keep it juicy. Once it's cooked to your liking, remove from the oven and wrap in foil while you get on with the gravy.
5. Pour any juices from the tin into a medium non-stick saucepan and turn the heat to medium. Sprinkle over the flour and stir well, cooking for 1 minute. Add the beef stock slowly, stirring.
6. Bring to the boil, then reduce the heat to low and simmer for 10–15 minutes, until thickened.
7. Serve with lots of greens and the dauphinoise potatoes, opposite.

Happier, Healthier, Tastier!

Dauphinoise potatoes Ⓥ

800g potatoes (such as Maris Piper) peeled
3 rosemary or thyme sprigs
250g reduced-fat crème fraiche
50ml semi-skimmed milk
50g reduced-fat Cheddar, grated
1 tsp Dijon mustard
Freshly ground black pepper

Per serving: Carbs: 19g | Calories: 177 | Fat: 8.4g | Protein: 17.2g

1. Preheat the oven to 160°C/140°C Fan/Gas 4.
2. Slice the potatoes into discs about the thickness of a £1 coin.
3. Boil the potatoes and rosemary or thyme sprigs in a large saucepan over a high heat, with the lid on, for around 5 minutes until the potatoes are almost cooked through but not falling apart.
4. In a large bowl, mix the the crème fraiche, milk, half of the cheese, Dijon mustard and a good grinding of black pepper.
5. Drain the potatoes and add to the bowl, carefully folding them through the sauce.
6. Spoon this mixture into a medium-sized oven dish, spreading the potatoes as evenly as possible, then top with the remaining cheese and another few grinds of black pepper.
7. Bake in the oven for around 40 minutes, until the cheese is melted and turning golden and the potatoes are cooked.

MAKES 12 (2 PER PERSON)

Yorkshire puddings Ⓥ

6 tsp vegetable oil
100g plain flour
2 eggs
100ml semi-skimmed milk

Per serving: Carbs: 19.1g | Calories: 201 | Fat: 10.4g | Protein: 7.7g

1. Preheat the oven to 230°C/ 210°C Fan/Gas 8.
2. Grab a muffin tin and divide the oil between the twelve holes. The oil is very important as it will help the puddings to puff up beautifully. Pop the tray in the oven for 5 minutes to get the oil really hot.
3. Grab a large bowl and beat the plain flour with the eggs, until smooth.
4. Slowly add the milk, whisking constantly, until a smooth batter forms with no lumps.
5. Pour the batter into a Pyrex jug and carefully remove the muffin tin from the oven.
6. Pour an even amount of batter into each hole (you'll probably need slightly less than you think as they do puff up a lot).
7. Bake the puddings in the oven for 20 minutes. It's very important not to open the oven door while they are cooking, as you need a steady heat for the duration of the cooking time and opening the door will cause the temperature to drop and stop them from puffing up nicely.

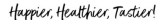

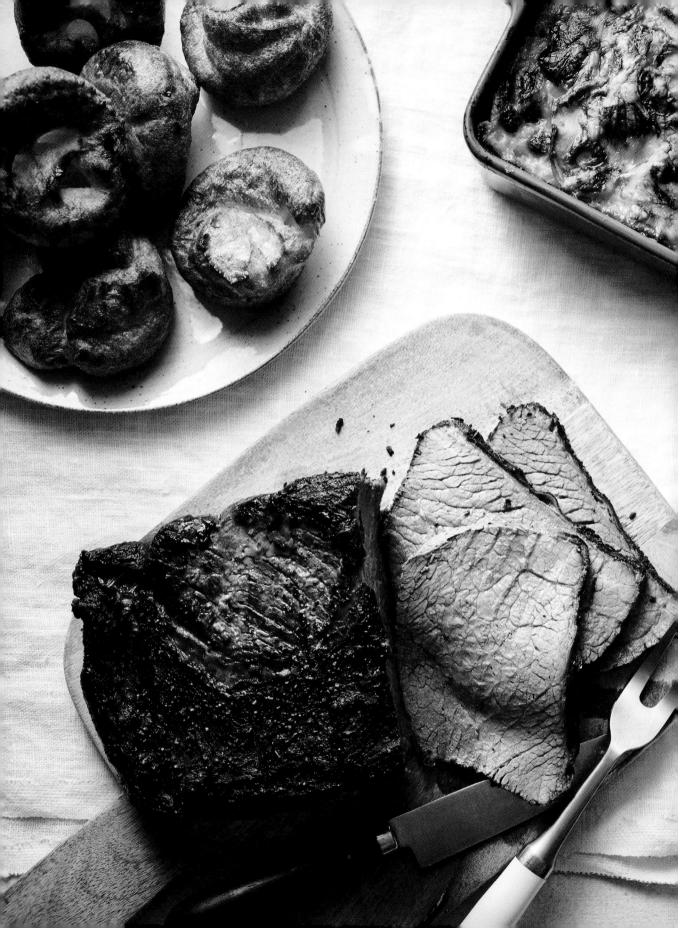

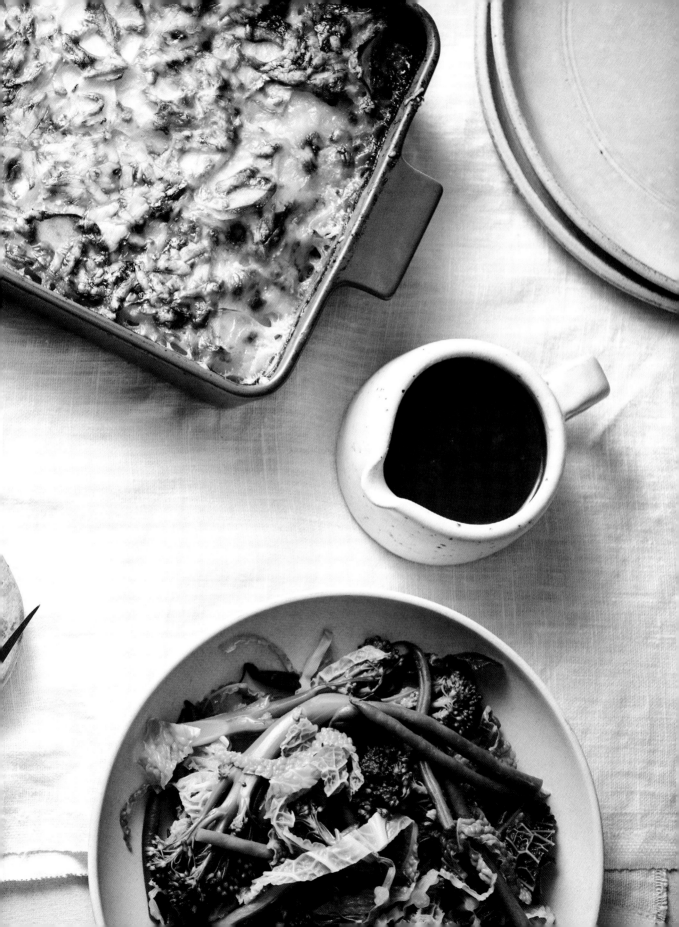

BBQ Feast

I'm up for a BBQ at any time of year. I just love it that most of the food here can be prepared in advance, ready to serve or to cook over the hot coals at the last minute. Nothing tastes better than eating char-grilled meat, fish or vegetables outside on a warm, sunny day, and nothing smells better than the aroma of wood smoke. This feast is so delicious and super healthy.

Healthy burgers

500g lean beef mince
1 egg, beaten
1 tsp dried Italian herbs
4 reduced-fat Cheddar slices
4 burger buns
4 tbsp tomato ketchup
4 tbsp light mayonnaise
Sliced lettuce, to serve
1 tomato, sliced
½ red onion, peeled and sliced
Sea salt
Freshly ground black pepper

Per serving: Carbs: 28.1g | Calories: 378 | Fat: 26.4g | Protein: 42.6g

1. In a large bowl, combine the beef mince with the egg and herbs and season well with sea salt and black pepper. Mix for a couple of minutes, until fully incorporated, then shape into four patties.
2. Place the burgers on the BBQ for around 5 minutes on each side, until cooked through.
3. Add the cheese slices on top of the patties and allow them to melt. Lightly toast the insides of your burger buns on the BBQ.
4. Mix the ketchup and mayonnaise, spread half on the bases of the burgers, then add the lettuce, the burger patties, the tomato and red onion. Spoon over the remaining sauce and finish with the burger-bun tops.

Potato salad Ⓥ

700g new potatoes, halved
3 tbsp light mayonnaise
3 tbsp fat-free yoghurt
2 tbsp reduced-fat crème fraîche
1 heaped tsp wholegrain mustard
1 bunch of spring onions, trimmed and very finely sliced
½ punnet fresh cress
Chives, very finely chopped, for sprinkling
Sea salt
Freshly ground black pepper

Per serving: Carbs: 18.6g | Calories: 112 | Fat: 2.6g | Protein: 2.6g

1. Boil the potatoes in salted water for around 10 minutes, until just cooked, then drain.
2. Meanwhile, mix the mayonnaise, yoghurt, crème fraîche and mustard in a small bowl.
3. While the potatoes are still warm, toss them together with the mayonnaise dressing, making sure they are well coated in the creamy sauce.
4. Season well with sea salt and black pepper, then toss through the spring onions. Sprinkle with cress and chopped chives, to serve.

Happier, Healthier, Tastier!

Grilled corn (v)

4 corn cobs
100g low-fat spread
1 garlic clove, finely grated
Sea salt
Freshly ground black pepper

Per serving: Carbs: 17.5g | Calories: 103 | Fat: 2.2g | Protein: 2.7g

1. To stop the corn from burning and to help it steam, place the cobs in a bowl of water to soak for 25–30 minutes, then drain the excess water and place each cob on a sheet of foil large enough to wrap it in.
2. Mix the spread with the garlic and season with sea salt and black pepper, then brush over the cobs.
3. Wrap the cobs up and cook on the BBQ for 25–30 minutes, turning now and again. Serve with the delicious, melted juices.

Harissa salmon skewers

4 × 130g skinless salmon fillets
4 tbsp harissa paste
2 red onions, peeled and cut into wedges, keeping the root intact
Fat-free yoghurt, to serve
Lime wedges, to serve
Sea salt

Per serving: Carbs: 4g | Calories: 281 | Fat: 13g | Protein: 39g

1. Cut the salmon into large chunks (there should be four to five pieces per skewer) then add to a small bowl, along with the harissa paste, and toss to coat.
2. Grab some metal or soaked wooden skewers and thread with a piece of salmon, followed by a wedge of red onion; keep going until you've filled four skewers with all the salmon and onion wedges.
3. Season with salt and place on the BBQ to cook for 10 minutes, turning halfway, until cooked through.
4. Serve with the yoghurt and lime wedges.

Happier, Healthier, Tastier!

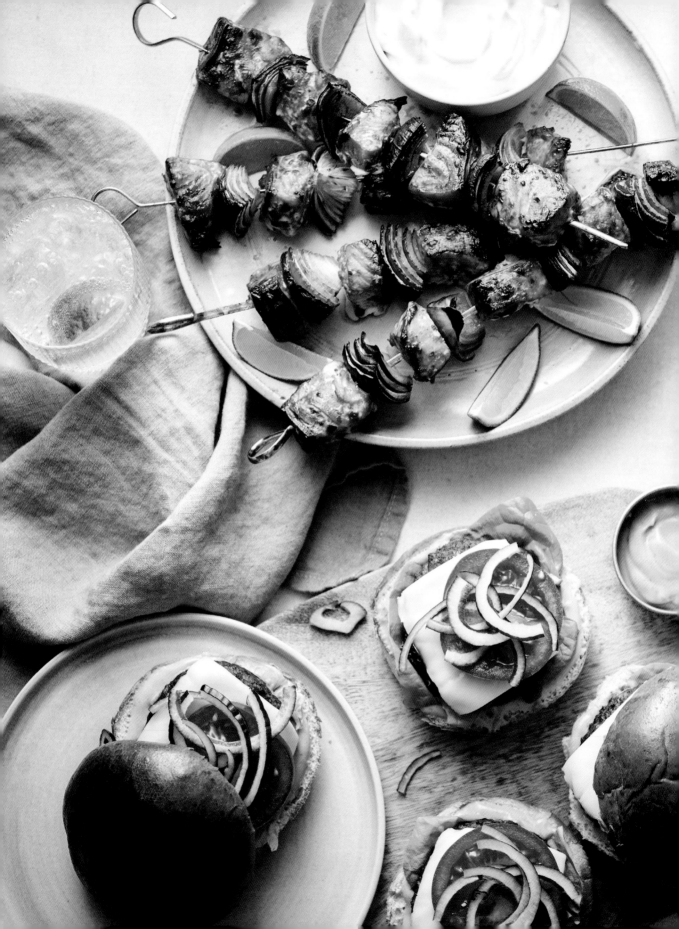

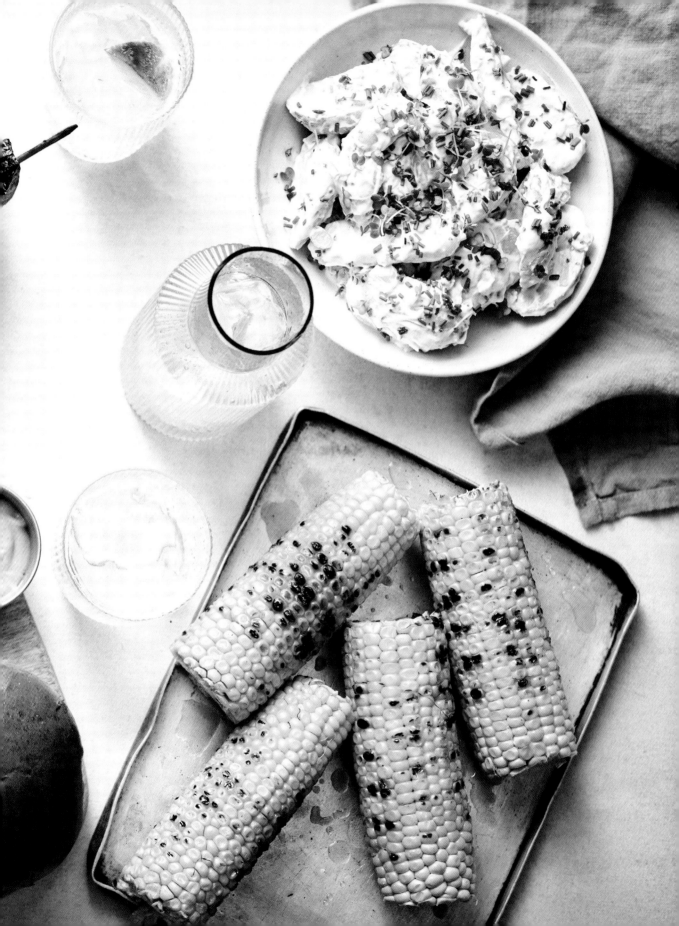

Steak with Chimichurri Sauce

SERVES 4

This is the real special-occasion-blowout dinner for all of you who love your red meat. For sensational results you need to buy the best, most tender piece of steak you can find, but it will still be a lot less pricey than eating it in a restaurant. Served with low-fat, golden crispy potatoes, lightly spiced green chimichurri and salad, it's insanely good.

Seared steak

1kg steak (a chateaubriand or côte de boeuf)
1 tsp olive oil
1 tbsp salted butter
5 garlic cloves, unpeeled but lightly crushed with the palm of your hand
Sea salt
Freshly ground black pepper

Per serving: Carbs: 0g | Calories: 295 | Fat: 21.6g | Protein: 24.6g

1. Preheat the oven to 220°C/200°C Fan/Gas 7. Line a baking tray with foil.
2. Rub the steak with the olive oil and season well with sea salt and black pepper.
3. Heat a medium, heavy-based, non-stick frying pan over a very high heat and, once smoking, add the steak. Leave it for around 3–4 minutes, until it has formed a lovely, crusty sear.
4. Flip and do the same on the other side. Depending on how large your steak is, it may be worth also searing the sides or the fat if it is thick.
5. Add the butter and garlic cloves to the pan, then spoon over the steak as the butter melts, for a couple of minutes.
6. Transfer the steak to the lined baking tray and cook in the oven for around 17 minutes for medium–rare. Test the steak by pressing it: if it is very squidgy, then it is very rare; you want a bit of bounce, but not too much. Remove from the oven and leave to rest, wrapped tightly in foil, for 20 minutes.

Happier, Healthier, Tastier!

Crispy potatoes VE

1kg new potatoes, unpeeled
2 tbsp olive oil
Sea salt

Per serving: Carbs: 42.8g | Calories: 247 | Fat: 7.5g | Protein: 4.3g

1. Cook the potatoes in boiling water, then drain and leave to steam-dry.
2. Grab a baking tray and add the oil and potatoes, tossing to coat. Season well with sea salt.
3. Using a potato masher, gently squish the potatoes, just so the skins break slightly.
4. Bake in the oven (temperature as for the steak, above) for 40–45 minutes, until crispy.

Chimichurri VE

3 tbsp olive oil
½ bunch of fresh coriander, finely chopped
½ bunch of fresh flat-leaf parsley, finely chopped
Handful of fresh mint, finely chopped
1 tbsp white wine vinegar
½ tsp dried chilli flakes
½ garlic clove, finely grated
Sea salt
Freshly ground black pepper

Per serving: Carbs: 0g | Calories: 90 | Fat: 10.1g | Protein: 0g

1. Combine all the ingredients in a bowl and stir well.

Rocket and Parmesan salad

2 tbsp olive oil
1 tbsp balsamic vinegar
80g rocket leaves
10 cherry tomatoes, halved
80g Parmesan, shaved with a speed peeler
Balsamic glaze, for drizzling

Per serving: Carbs: 2.4g | Calories: 145 | Fat: 11.8g | Protein: 7.6g

1. Combine the olive oil and balsamic vinegar, then toss through the rocket leaves and cherry tomatoes.
2. Top with the Parmesan shavings and drizzle with balsamic glaze.

Happier, Healthier, Tastier!

Desserts

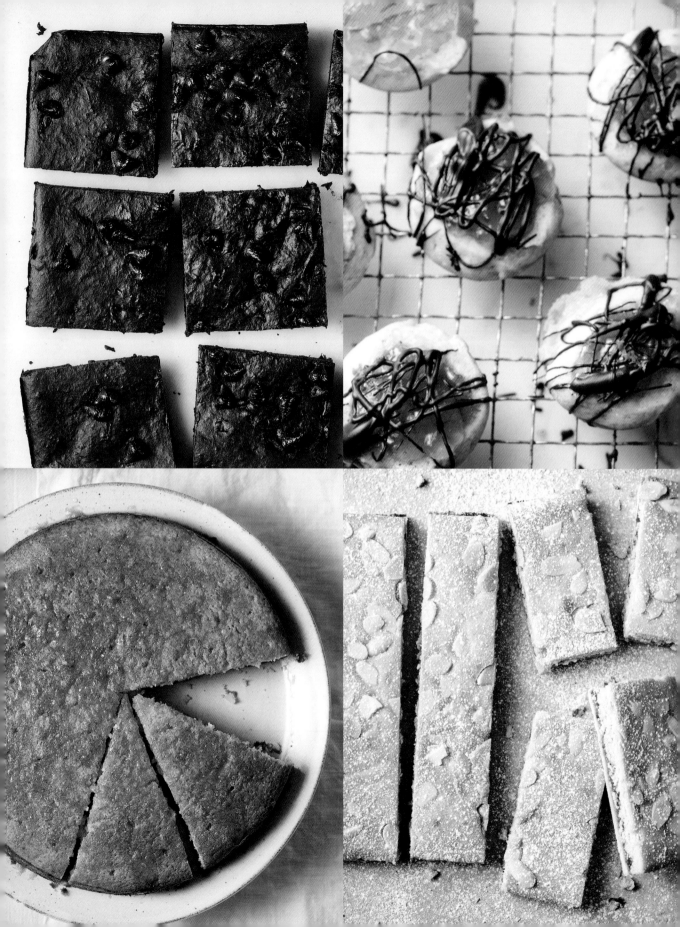

Ultimate Protein Chocolate Cake
Lemon Drizzle Cake
Mini Millionaire Shortbreads
Biscoff Cheesecake
Vegan Fudge Brownies
Jaffa Cakes
Baked Churros
Salted Peanut Chocolate Bars
Baked Custard Tarts
Peanut Butter Pie
Bakewell Tart Traybake
Oreo Brownies
Protein Birthday Cake
Rhubarb and Apple Crumble

Ultimate Protein Chocolate Cake Ⓥ

Per serving:

Carbs: 22g

Calories: 241

Fat: 15g

Protein: 19.3g

A slice of this awesome chocolate cake might seem super indulgent, but – at less than a whopping 19 grams of protein and 250 calories per slice – it won't affect your fitness goals. Tinned black beans might seem like a surprising addition, but take my word for it – they make the cake really moist and add protein and fibre, making it super healthy, too.

SERVES 10
60g dark chocolate
30g white chocolate
1 × 400g tin black beans, drained and rinsed
4 large eggs
90g cocoa powder (unsweetened)
4 tbsp ground almonds
3 tbsp golden caster sugar
1 tbsp zero-calorie maple syrup
4 tbsp granulated sweetener
60g low-fat spread, melted
2 tsp vanilla extract
1 tsp baking powder
½ tsp bicarbonate of soda
300g extra-light cream cheese
50g chocolate protein powder
1 tbsp powdered sweetener

1. Start by melting the dark chocolate in a bowl in the microwave for 30-second blasts, until smooth. In another bowl, do the same with the white chocolate.
2. Line a baking tray with non-stick baking paper. Pour over the dark chocolate and pour evenly over the tray to form a roughly shaped, thin sheet of chocolate. Drop dollops of the white chocolate over the top and swirl with a toothpick to marble the two together. Refrigerate while you make the cake.
3. Preheat the oven to 180°C/160°C Fan/Gas 4. Line an 18cm round cake tin around the base and sides with non-stick baking paper.
4. Place the black beans, eggs, 60g of the cocoa powder, ground almonds, golden caster sugar, maple syrup, granulated sweetener, low-fat spread, vanilla extract, baking powder and bicarbonate of soda in a food processor and blitz, until smooth.
5. Pour the mixture into the prepared cake tin and bake for around 30–35 minutes, until it is cooked and the surface springs back when pressed.
6. While the cake is cooling, prepare the topping by whipping together the remaining 30g cocoa powder, cream cheese, protein powder and powdered sweetener.
7. Once the cake has cooled, top with the chocolate frosting. Break the chilled chocolate sheet into randomly sized shards and stick into the top of the cake at different angles.

Happier, Healthier, Tastier!

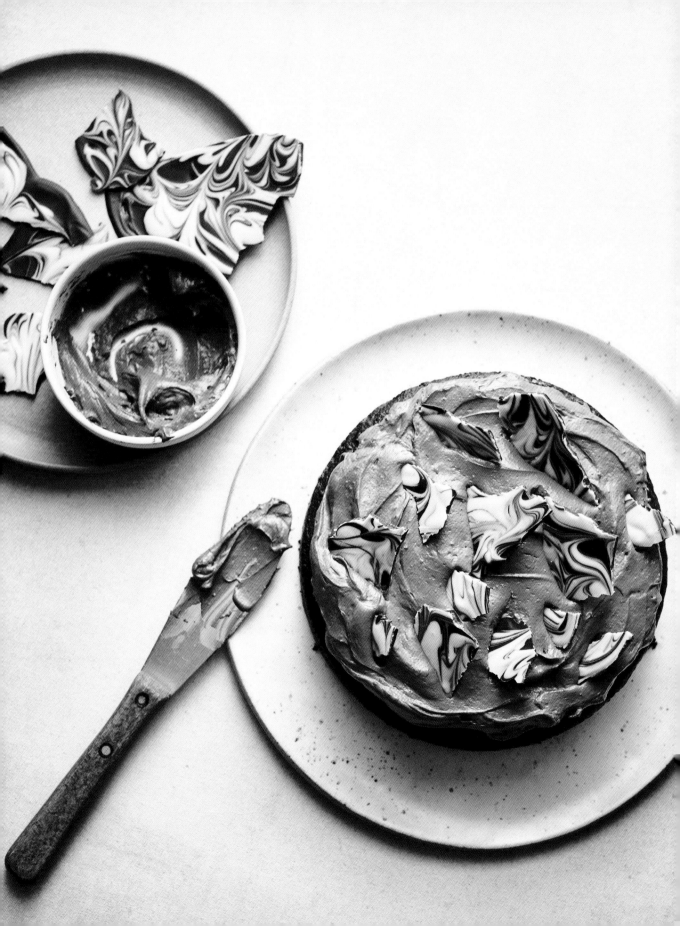

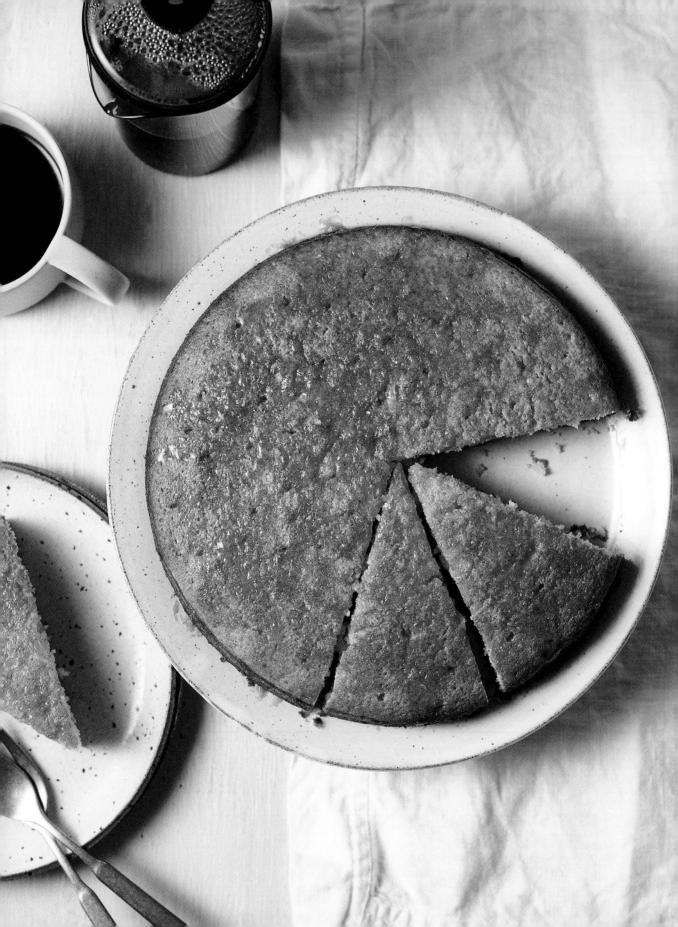

Lemon Drizzle Cake ⓥ

Per serving:

Carbs: 14.3g

Calories: 124

Fat: 4g

Protein: 6.5g

You don't have to go without your favourite cakes just because you're on a healthy-eating regime. The good news is that a slice of this deliciously moist lemon drizzle cake is so low in carbs and fat that you can treat yourself without worrying about the calories.

SERVES 8

Low-calorie cooking spray
6 large eggs, separated
3 lemons (juice of 3, zest of 2)
100g granulated sweetener
   plus 2 tsp
1 tbsp vanilla extract
150g self-raising flour
1 tsp baking powder
1 tbsp zero-calorie maple syrup

1. Preheat the oven to 180°C/160°C Fan/Gas 4. Grease a 20cm cake tin with low-calorie spray and line with non-stick baking paper.
2. Place the egg whites in a mixing bowl and whisk, until they have stiffened and formed peaks when the whisk is pulled up.
3. In another large bowl, whisk the egg yolks, the juice and zest of 1 lemon, the 100g of sweetener and the vanilla extract, until nearly doubled in size. It might help to use an electric whisk for these steps.
4. Sift half the flour into the egg-yolk mixture, along with the baking powder. Using a large metal spoon, gently fold the flour through the egg.
5. Add half of the beaten egg white and the remaining flour to the yolk mixture and fold together. Now add the rest of the egg white and fold, until you have a smooth cake mix. By adding each ingredient in stages and gently folding, you'll end up with a lighter sponge.
6. Pour the mixture into the cake tin and bake for 35–40 minutes. A cocktail stick inserted into the centre of the cake should come out clean when it's done.
7. While the cake is baking, place the remaining lemon juice, the remaining lemon zest, maple syrup and the 2 teaspoons of granulated sweetener in a small saucepan and warm over a low heat, stirring until the sweetener dissolves and the mixture has reduced slightly without boiling.
8. Once baked, remove the cake from the oven and place the tin on a wire rack.
9. Prick the top of the cake all over with a cocktail stick and pour over the warmed lemon syrup. Leave the cake to soak up the syrup.

Happier, Healthier, Tastier!

Mini Millionaire Shortbreads ⓥ

Per shortbread:

Carbs: 20g

Calories: 181

Fat: 10g

Protein: 1.6g

Who says you can't treat yourself on your fitness journey? If you're working out, eating healthily and feeling better, give yourself a well-earned reward and brighten up your day with one of these gorgeous mini shortbreads. Your family and friends will love them, too. Make this vegan by swapping the milk and dark chocolate for vegan varieties.

MAKES 14
140g gluten-free plain flour
95g low-fat spread
1 tbsp caster sugar
120g soft pitted dates
1 tbsp cashew nut butter
3 tbsp coconut oil, melted
1 tbsp zero-calorie maple syrup
2 tsp vanilla extract
½ tsp sea salt
3 tbsp semi-skimmed milk
150g dark chocolate

1. Preheat the oven to 180°C/160°C Fan/Gas 4. Line a 20cm square tin with non-stick baking paper.
2. Place the flour, low-fat spread and caster sugar in a food processor and pulse, until you have a smooth dough. Tip into the prepared tin and press down to flatten. Prick the shortbread base with a fork and transfer to the oven to bake for 23–25 minutes, until hard and beginning to crisp. The shortbread should still have a pale colour to it. Leave to cool completely.
3. To make the caramel layer, place the dates, cashew nut butter, half the coconut oil, maple syrup, vanilla extract and salt to a food processor.
4. Add the milk to a small saucepan and bring to a simmer. Remove from the heat and add 2 tablespoons to the food processor.
5. Blitz, until you have a smooth paste. Add the remaining milk if the mixture is too thick and sticky to blend properly.
6. Spoon the caramel layer over the shortbread. Spread evenly and place in the fridge for 30 minutes to cool and set.
7. Melt the chocolate and remaining coconut oil together in the microwave in 30-second bursts, then pour over the caramel layer. Return to the fridge and allow all the layers to finish setting before removing from the tin and slicing.

Happier, Healthier, Tastier!

Biscoff Cheesecake

Per serving:

Carbs: 27g

Calories: 230

Fat: 9.4g

Protein: 9.8g

You can make this no-cook creamy cheesecake in under twenty minutes and then leave it in the fridge to chill for two hours or even overnight. At only 230 calories per slice, you don't have to worry about treating yourself when you crave something sweet.

SERVES 8

Low-calorie cooking spray
180g Lotus Biscoff biscuits,
    plus 3 extra for the topping
55g low-fat spread, melted
60ml lukewarm water
9g powdered gelatin
400g extra-light cream cheese
250g low-fat yoghurt
2 tbsp Lotus Biscoff spread
1 tbsp granulated sweetener
2 tsp vanilla extract

1. Lightly grease a 20cm cake tin with cooking spray, then line with non-stick baking paper.
2. In a food processor, blitz the 180g biscuits until they reach a fine crumb consistency, then combine with the low-fat spread.
3. Press the mixture into the bottom of the cake tin and pop in the fridge.
4. Pour the water into a small, heatproof bowl and sprinkle over the gelatin. Mix together and set aside for a few minutes, until it has started to thicken. Heat the mixture in the microwave on low for about 30 seconds, until the mixture has liquified but is not hot.
5. Place the cream cheese, yoghurt and Biscoff spread in a bowl or stand mixer with a paddle attachment and beat for 2 minutes, until the mixture is light and fluffy. Continue mixing while you slowly pour in the gelatin mixture, until smooth.
6. Add the granulated sweetener and vanilla and beat again until light and smooth. Tip the mixture into the chilled base and spread evenly. Chill in the fridge for at least 2 hours before crumbling the extra biscuits on top.

Happier, Healthier, Tastier!

Vegan Fudge Brownies (VE)

Per serving:

Carbs: 11.2g

Calories: 127

Fat: 1g

Protein: 3.7g

You're going to be knocked out by this insanely good recipe for vegan brownies. And they're so quick and easy to make in a food processor. Serve them to your family and friends and they won't be able to tell the difference.

MAKES 9

250g ripe bananas

70g apple sauce

1 tsp caramel flavouring

60g vegan cocoa powder

1 tbsp granulated sweetener

35g vegan chocolate protein powder

½ tsp fine sea salt

50g vegan chocolate chips, plus 15g extra for topping

½ tsp fine sea salt

1. Preheat the oven to 190°C/170°C Fan/Gas 5.
2. Line a 20cm square brownie tin with non-stick baking paper, leaving a little extra sticking out on either side, to help with lifting out.
3. Place the bananas, apple sauce, caramel flavouring, cocoa powder, sweetener, protein powder and salt in a food processor and blitz, until you have a smooth batter.
4. Mix in the 50g of chocolate chips by hand and spoon the batter into the tin evenly, then scatter the remaining chocolate chips over the top, pressing them down.
5. Bake in the oven for 20 minutes, then remove from oven and leave to cool slightly before lifting out and cutting into 9 squares.

Happier, Healthier, Tastier!

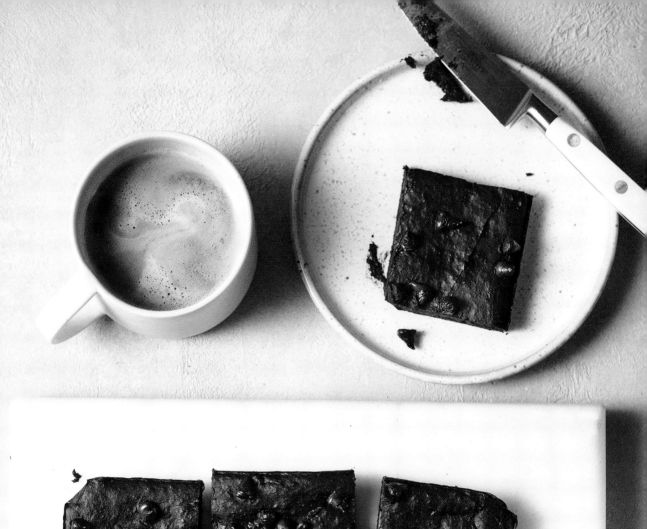
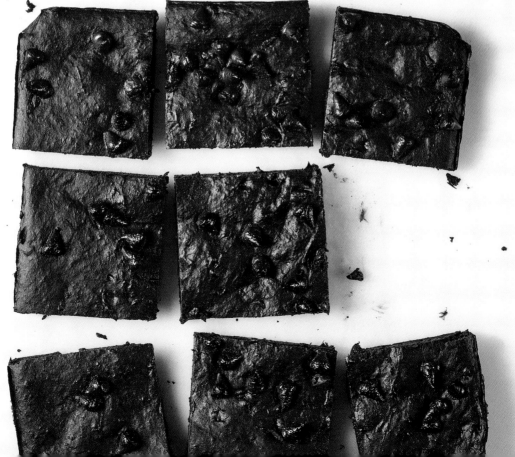

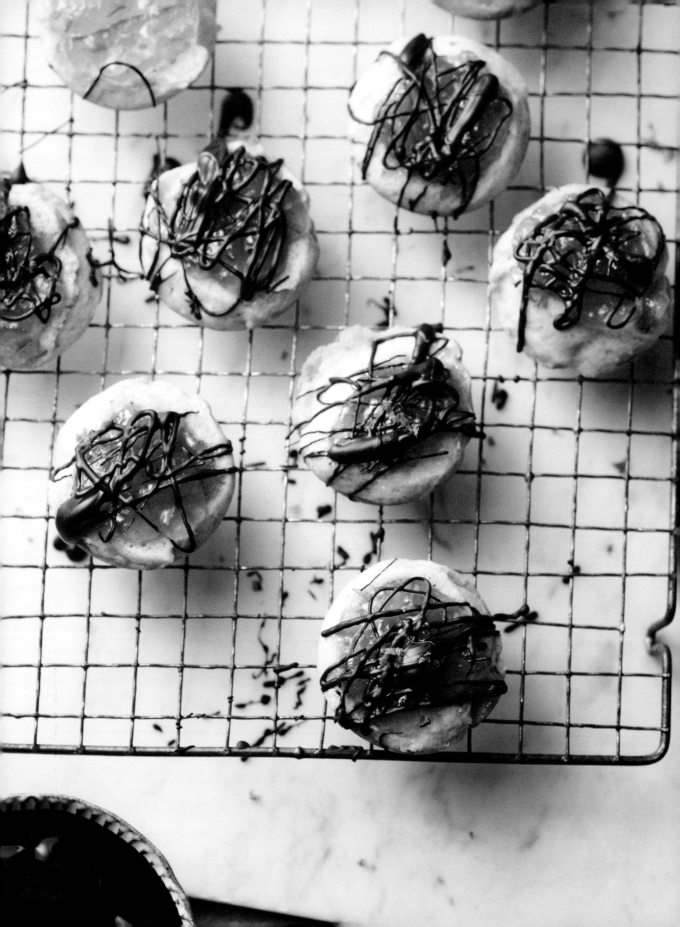

Jaffa Cakes ⓥ

Per cake:

Carbs: 17.8g

Calories: 131

Fat: 5.9g

Protein: 2.8g

If these don't make your mouth water, I don't know what will. Homemade Jaffa cakes are so yummy and much healthier than shop-bought ones. If you're into baking, this is a great way to spend an hour on a rainy afternoon at the weekend. Your family or friends will thank you for it.

MAKES 12

130g plain flour
½ tsp baking powder
¼ tsp sea salt
3 tbsp low-fat spread, melted
3 tbsp zero-calorie maple syrup
1 tsp vanilla extract
1 tbsp golden caster sugar
20ml semi-skimmed milk
Low-calorie cooking spray
Zest of ½ orange
90g no-added-sugar orange marmalade
150g dark chocolate, melted

1. Preheat the oven to 180°C/160°C Fan/Gas 4.
2. In a large bowl, sift the flour, baking powder and salt together. Add the melted low-fat spread, maple syrup, vanilla extract, caster sugar and milk, and mix together to form a smooth batter.
3. Spray a 12-hole cupcake tin with low-calorie cooking spray, then add 2 teaspoons of batter to each of the holes.
4. Bake in the oven for 10–12 minutes, until lightly golden, then remove and leave to cool on a wire rack. Once cool, remove the sponges from the tin.
5. Mix half the orange zest through the marmalade, then place a teaspoon of marmalade in the centre of each sponge base, using a knife to flatten the top of the dollop.
6. Drizzle the melted chocolate over the tops of the cakes to cover the marmalade, then top with a light sprinkling of the remaining orange zest, before chilling in the fridge for 30 minutes.

Happier, Healthier, Tastier!

Baked Churros ⓥ

Per churro:

Carbs: 22.9g

Calories: 207

Fat: 10.5g

Protein: 3.7g

Traditional Spanish churros are fried in hot oil, making them a high-calorie dessert or treat. These, however, baked in the oven, are much healthier and lower in fat, so you can enjoy more of them! Dusted with cinnamon and sugar they're as good as they look.

MAKES AROUND 20
200ml water
90g low-fat spread
20g golden caster sugar, plus
  2 tbsp for dusting
100g plain flour
1 large egg, beaten
2 tsp vanilla extract
2 tsp ground cinammon
Low-calorie cooking spray

1. Preheat the oven to 180°C/160°C Fan/Gas 4 and line a flat baking tray with non-stick baking paper.
2. Place the water, low-fat spread and sugar in a medium non-stick saucepan. Bring to the boil, then turn off the heat.
3. Add the flour and stir constantly, until you have a smooth paste. Remove the pan and leave to cool for 2 minutes.
4. Add the egg and vanilla extract and, working quickly, mix them in. Keep mixing, until you have a smooth, shiny dough.
5. Spoon the dough into a piping bag with a star-shaped nozzle and pipe small sausage shapes on to the prepared baking tray. It should make around twenty churros.
6. Bake in the oven for 35–40 minutes, until the pastry has puffed up and turned golden.
7. In a shallow bowl, mix the cinnamon with the remaining sugar. Spray the churros whilst warm with low-calorie cooking spray, then dip them in the cinnamon sugar. Serve with your favourite chocolate sauce.

Happier, Healthier, Tastier!

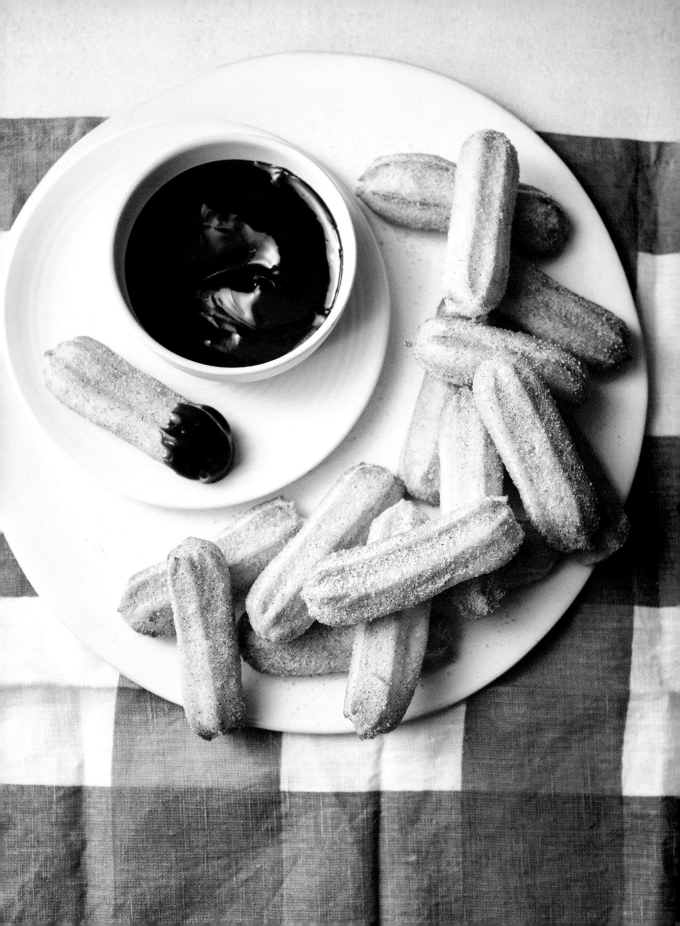

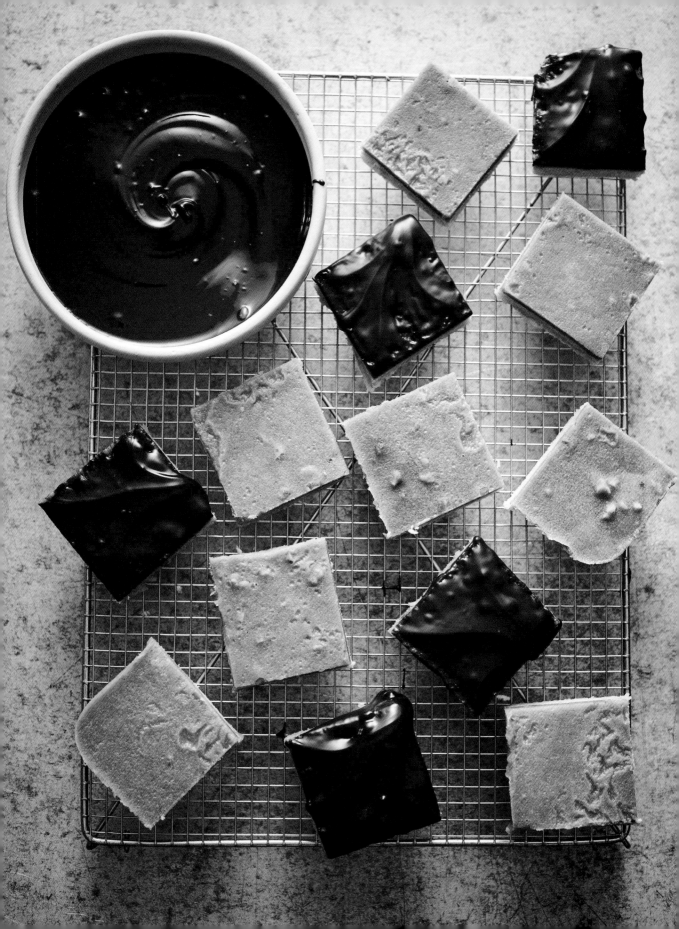

Salted Peanut Chocolate Bars 🅥🅔

Per bar:

Carbs: 7.9g

Calories: 186

Fat: 14g

Protein: 9.6g

To make these delish vegan bars you use a mixture of almond and coconut flour – both are available in most health-food stores and large supermarkets. At only 186 calories per bar, you can eat one as a post workout treat or pop one into your lunch box.

MAKES 16

220g almond flour
1 tsp fine sea salt, plus extra, to serve
2 tbsp coconut flour
120g coconut oil, melted
160g zero-calorie maple syrup
50g smooth peanut butter
50g chunky peanut butter
1 tsp vanilla extract
200g vegan chocolate chips

1. Preheat the oven to 180°C/160°C Fan/Gas 4 and line a small brownie tin with non-stick baking paper.
2. Combine the almond flour, half a teaspoon of salt and the coconut flour in a bowl. Add half the melted coconut oil and half the maple syrup, until you have a smooth paste. Tip the mixture into the prepared tin and smooth the top.
3. Bake for 12–14 minutes, until lightly browned, then remove from the oven and leave in the tin to cool on a wire rack.
4. In a small saucepan, combine the peanut butters, the remaining coconut oil and maple syrup, vanilla extract and the remaining salt. Gently warm over a low heat for 3–5 minutes, until melted and combined. Leave to cool slightly before pouring over the shortbread. Smooth over and chill in the fridge for 30 minutes.
5. Once cooled, carefully lift out of the tray and cut in half lengthways, then slice into 16 bars.
6. Melt the chocolate chips and dip each bar, upside down, to coat. Place the bars on a wire rack and sprinkle with a few flecks of sea salt. Transfer the rack to the fridge to set the chocolate for a few minutes before enjoying.

Happier, Healthier, Tastier!

Baked Custard Tarts ⓥ

Per tart:

Carbs: 27.3g

Calories: 242

Fat: 9.7g

Protein: 7g

My creamy custard tarts are a revelation! Most of the ones you buy are loaded with carbs and fat, but by using light puff pastry, skimmed milk and granulated sweetener instead of sugar, I've created a delicious, low-calorie alternative that everyone will enjoy.

MAKES 8

1 tbsp plain flour
1 × 375g pack ready-rolled light puff pastry
1 tbsp ground cinnamon, plus ½ tsp
½ tbsp ground nutmeg
Low-calorie cooking spray
450ml skimmed milk
3 tbsp cornflour
4½ tbsp granulated sweetener
2 egg yolks
1 tsp vanilla extract

1. Preheat the oven to 200°C/180°C Fan/Gas 6.
2. Dust a work surface with the flour. Roll out the pastry sheet and, using a sieve, sprinkle it with the ground cinnamon and nutmeg. Roll up the sheet, leading with one of the longer sides and slice the roll into 8 equal pieces.
3. Place each piece, sliced side up (so you can see the rings of the pastry) and push down with the palm of your hand. Take a dusted rolling pin and roll each piece into a 10cm disc.
4. Lightly grease a muffin tin with low-calorie spray. Lay each pastry disc inside a muffin hole, pressing them down into the bottom and smoothing up the sides.
5. Bake the pastry cases in the oven for 10–12 minutes, until crisp and golden.
6. Pour the milk into a medium-sized saucepan, slowly bring to a gentle simmer, then remove from the heat.
7. Add the cornflour, sweetener, egg yolks, vanilla and the half teaspoon cinnamon to a medium mixing bowl and beat together with a whisk.
8. Gradually whisk the milk into the egg mixture, bit by bit.
9. Transfer the mixture back to the pan and cook over a low heat – it should begin to thicken.
10. Pour the custard into the baked pastry cases, being careful not to overfill.
11. Pop the tarts back into the oven and bake for 16–18 minutes. Watch the tarts near the end of the cooking time to ensure they don't burn.
12. Remove from the oven and leave for 15 minutes to cool and set before enjoying.

Happier, Healthier, Tastier!

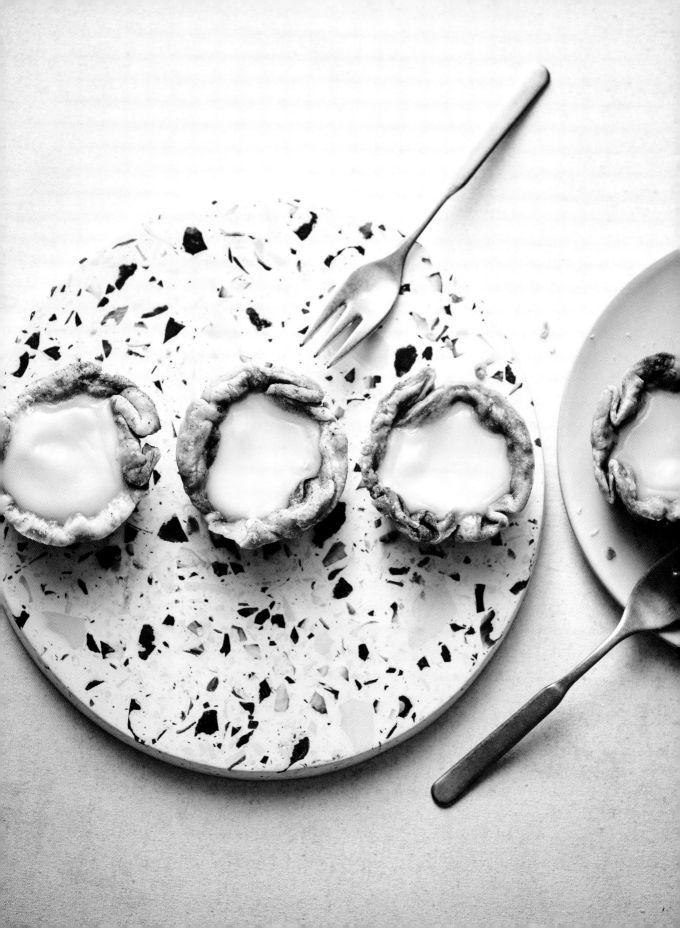

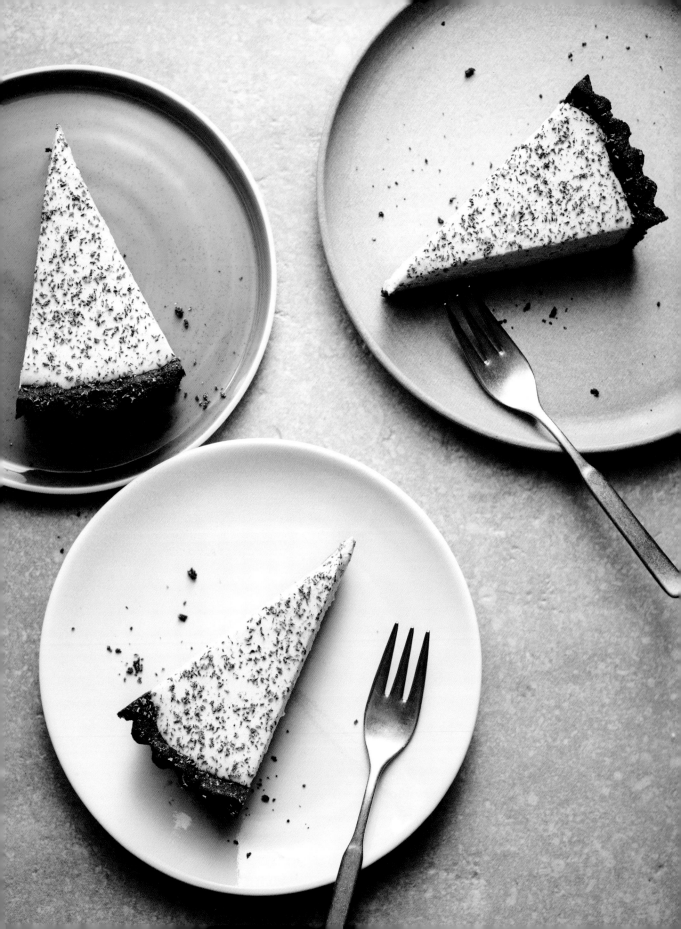

Peanut Butter Pie ⓥ

Per serving:

Carbs: 7g

Calories: 271

Fat: 21g

Protein: 12g

You've never tasted pie like this before! The base is made with almonds and coconut oil, and the creamy filling is flavoured with peanut butter. Nuts are so healthy, delicious and packed with protein, vitamins and minerals, making every slice a nutritious treat.

SERVES 10

Low-calorie cooking spray
230g almond flour
25g cocoa powder, unsweetened
60g coconut oil
160g zero-calorie maple syrup
1½ tbsp boiling water
2 tsp powdered gelatin
500g light cream cheese
3 tbsp smooth peanut butter
2 tsp vanilla extract
2 tbsp granulated sweetener
1 tbsp semi-skimmed milk

1. Preheat the oven to 180°C/160°C Fan/Gas 4. Lightly grease a 23cm pie tin (preferably with a removable base).
2. Place the almond flour, cocoa powder, coconut oil and half the maple syrup in a food processor and pulse, until the ingredients turn into a well-combined crumbly, sticky mix.
3. Press the base mixture into the pie tin and up the sides. Make sure to get an even coverage, pressing over any cracks. Prick the base with a fork and place it in the oven for 15 minutes, then remove and cool on a wire rack.
4. Pour the boiling water into a heatproof jug. Sprinkle the gelatin over the water and whisk with a fork, until dissolved. Set aside to cool.
5. To prepare the filling, combine the cream cheese, peanut butter, vanilla extract, sweetener and milk in a mixing bowl and beat with an electric whisk for 3–4 minutes, until light and the peanut butter is incorporated throughout.
6. Gradually beat in the gelatin mixture, until combined. Spoon the mixture into the prepared crust and refrigerate, until set (preferably overnight). Once set, slice and serve.

Happier, Healthier, Tastier!

Bakewell Tart Traybake ⓥ

Baking couldn't be easier when you use ready-rolled pastry and an all-in-one sponge-cake mixture. The prep takes under ten minutes and there's no fancy icing or decorations, making this is a quick take on an old-fashioned family favourite. Just what you've been waiting for.

Per bar:

Carbs: 23.7g

Calories: 192

Fat: 9.1g

Protein: 3.4g

MAKES 16–18 BARS

1 × 375g pack ready-rolled light shortcrust pastry
170g self-raising flour
130g low-fat spread
50g caster sugar
1 tbsp granulated sweetener
2 large eggs
1 tsp baking powder
½ tsp almond extract
2 tbsp semi-skimmed milk
6 tbsp reduced-sugar raspberry (or strawberry) jam
30g flaked almonds
1 tbsp icing sugar

1. Preheat the oven to 180°C/160°C Fan/Gas 4.
2. On a lightly floured surface, roll out the pastry and use it to to line the base of a rectangular brownie tin (length around 29cm).
3. In a large bowl, beat the self-raising flour, low-fat spread, caster sugar, granulated sweetener, eggs, baking powder, almond extract and milk, until smooth.
4. Spread the jam over the base of the pastry, then pour the batter on top.
5. Sprinkle over the flaked almonds and bake in the oven for around 25–30 minutes, until golden.
6. Leave to cool, then dust with icing sugar, cut into bars and serve.

Happier, Healthier, Tastier!

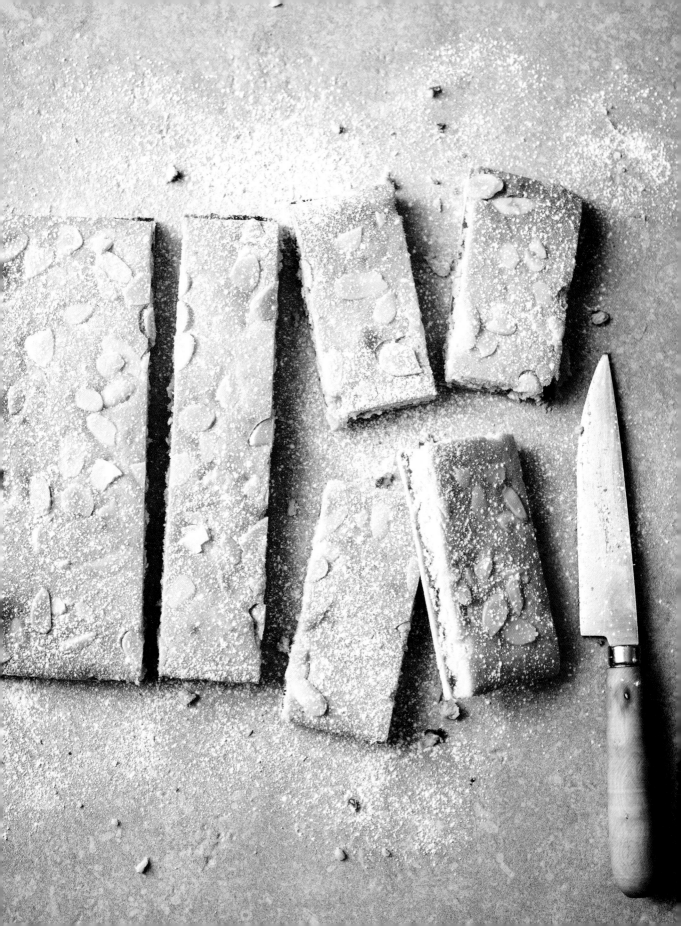

Oreo Brownies ⓥ

Per brownie:

Carbs: 18g

Calories: 149

Fat: 4g

Protein: 6g

You're going to be obsessed with these low-cal, low-fat, low-carb brownies. Not only are they unbelievably yummy, but they're made with healthy protein powder, yoghurt and oats. If you're a chocolate fanatic like me and love Oreos, they'll be your go-to daily treat.

MAKES 14

6 Oreos
10 Oreo Thins
160g instant oats
35g chocolate protein powder
180g low-fat thick yoghurt
130ml semi-skimmed milk
60g cocoa powder
50g granulated sweetener
1 tsp baking powder
1 egg
2 tsp vanilla extract
¼ tsp sea salt

1. Preheat the oven to 180°C/160°C Fan/Gas 4. Grease and line a baking tray with non-stick baking paper.
2. Grab two bowls and break the Oreos into chunks into one and the Oreo Thins into the other.
3. Place the remaining ingredients in a food processor and blitz, until smooth.
4. Pour the mixture into a bowl and stir through the Oreo chunks (not the Thins). Pour into the prepared baking tray, smooth the top and scatter over the crumbled Oreo Thins pieces.
5. Bake in the oven for 25–30 minutes, until the centre is just cooked.
6. Remove from the oven and leave to stand for 10 minutes before slicing.

Happier, Healthier, Tastier!

Protein Birthday Cake ⓥ

Bet you never thought such a delectable cake could give you 24 grams of protein per slice –and it's all in the low-cal vanilla frosting. How clever is that? Even if you've never baked before, you'll be the star of the birthday party with this amazing cake. For the finishing touch, just light the candles and make a wish.

Per serving:

Carbs: 23g

Calories: 295

Fat: 12g

Protein: 24g

SERVES 8

Low-calorie cooking spray
130g self-raising flour
2 tsp baking powder
130g vanilla protein powder
150g low-fat spread
30g caster sugar
50g granulated sweetener
4 medium eggs
½ tbsp semi-skimmed milk
5 tsp vanilla extract
350g extra-light cream cheese
1 tsp fine powdered sweetener
100g fat-free yoghurt
4 tsp rainbow sprinkles
10g white chocolate curls

1. Preheat the oven to 160°C/140°C Fan/Gas 4, then grease two 20cm round cake tins with the cooking spray and line the bases and sides with non-stick baking paper.
2. In a large bowl, sift the flour, baking powder and 100g of the protein powder together.
3. In another bowl, mix the low-fat spread, sugar and granulated sweetener, until smooth.
4. Add the eggs to the sugar mixture, one at a time and whisk for a few minutes, until you have a light mixture.
5. Add the milk and 3 teaspoons of the vanilla extract and mix again. Add to the dry ingredients and mix together, until you have a smooth cake batter.
6. Divide the mixture between the two prepared cake tins and bake in the oven for 30–35 minutes, until a skewer inserted into the centre of the sponges comes out clean.
7. While the sponges are baking, beat the cream cheese, remaining vanilla extract, fine powdered sweetener and the remaining protein powder. Add the yoghurt gradually, mixing, until you have a spreadable frosting that isn't too smooth – it needs to hold inside the cake. Leave to set in the fridge.
8. When the cakes are cooked, leave them on a wire rack to cool. Remove from the tins and top one layer with half the frosting, top with the second cake layer, then decorate with the remaining icing, rainbow sprinkles and white chocolate curls.

Happier, Healthier, Tastier!

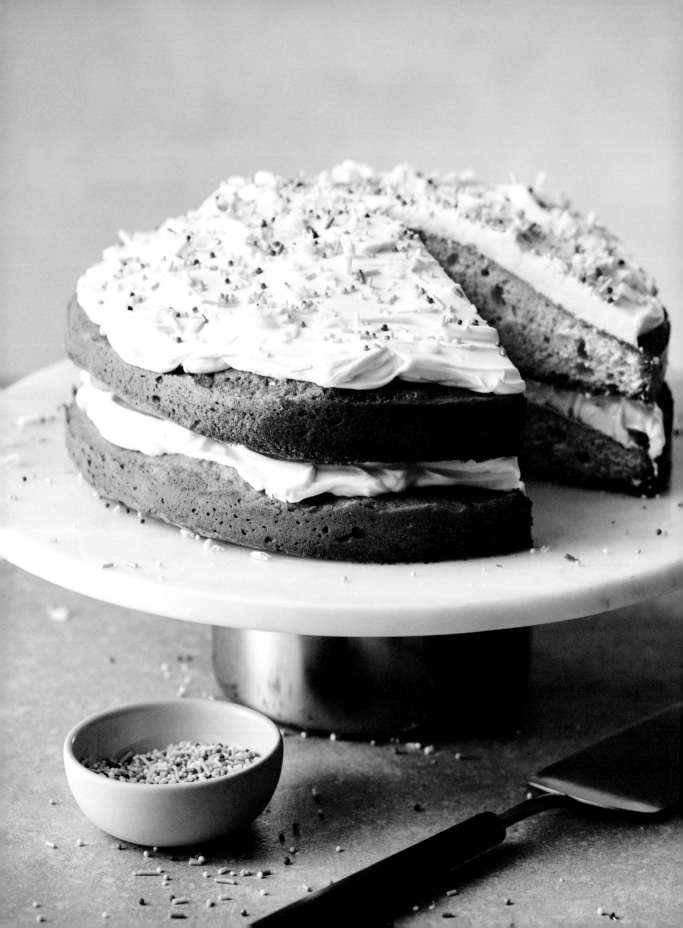

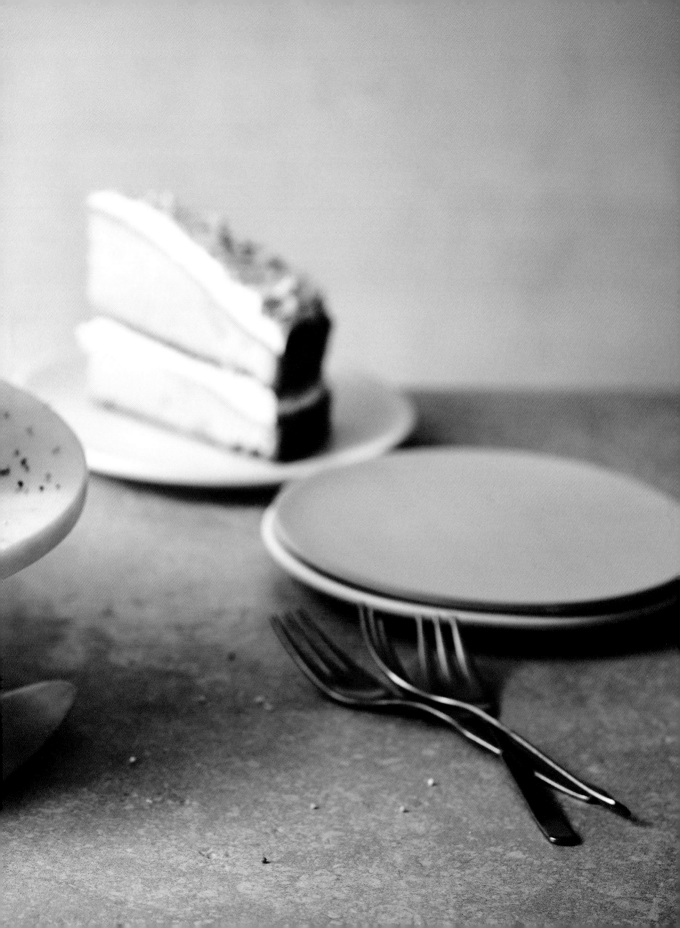

Rhubarb and Apple Crumble ⓥ

Everyone loves a fruit crumble but it's not always a very healthy choice. Look no further . . . my crumble is crunchy, golden and enriched with protein powder to make it super healthy. And at fewer than 230 calories per portion, you can serve it with custard, ice cream or a spoonful of half-fat crème fraîche. You can make this recipe vegan by swapping the low-fat spread and protein powder for vegan varieties.

Per serving:

Carbs: 35.8g

Calories: 227

Fat: 5.3g

Protein: 10.8g

SERVES 4

3 rhubarb sticks, sliced

2 red apples, peeled and cut into small cubes

1 tbsp golden caster sugar

100g plain flour

35g vanilla protein powder

2 tbsp demerara sugar

½ tsp ground cinnamon

2 tbsp low-fat spread

1. Preheat the oven to 200°C/180°C Fan/Gas 6.
2. Place the rhubarb, apples, caster sugar and a splash of water in a small non-stick saucepan, over a low–medium heat. Cover and cook for 10 minutes, until the fruit has softened but still has a bite to it. Divide the mixture between 4 small ramekins.
3. In a large bowl, mix the flour, protein powder, demerara sugar and cinnamon, until well combined. Rub the low-fat spread into the mixture with your fingers, until you reach a crumble consistency.
4. Spoon the crumble mixture over the stewed fruit and bake for around 20 minutes, until golden.
5. Serve with custard (optional).

Happier, Healthier, Tastier!

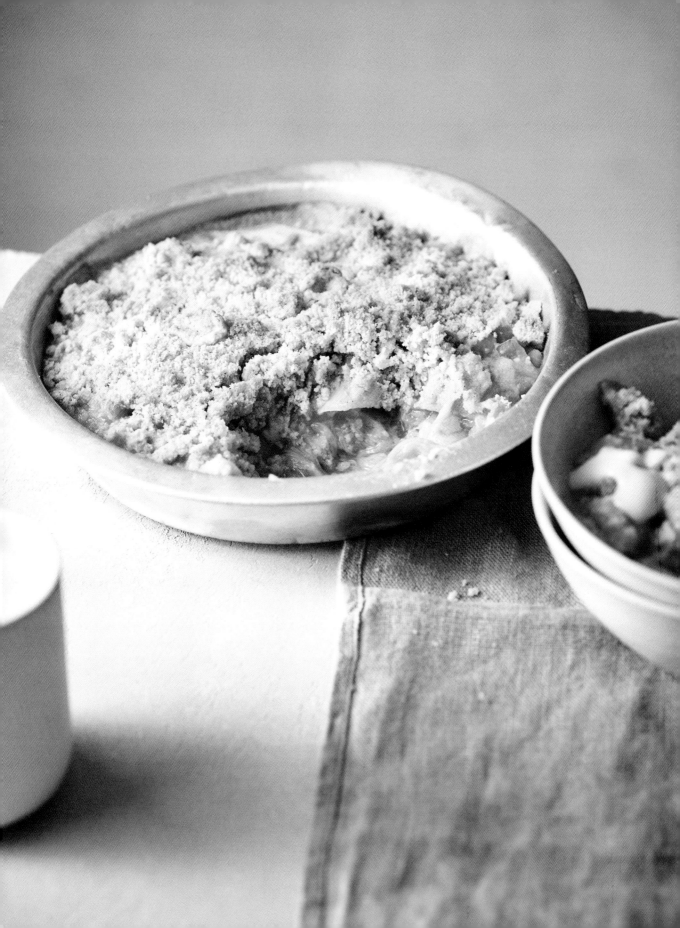

Index

Happier, Healthier, Tastier!

Happier, Healthier, Tastier!

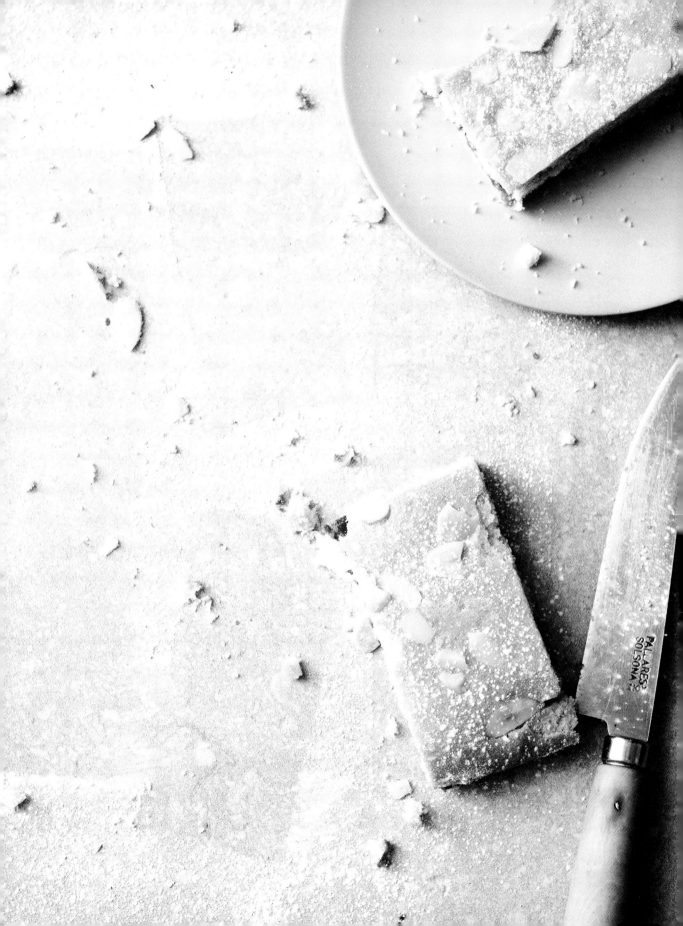

Happier, Healthier, Tastier!

Happier, Healthier, Tastier!

Happier, Healthier, Tastier!

Acknowledgements

Firstly, I'd like to thank the amazing, hardworking team at HarperCollins Publishers: Lydia, James, Georgina, Hattie and Lucy, and also Ollie and Heather. You really listened to what I wanted for my book and brought the vision to life.

To the shoot team who created the fantastic photos for the book: Anna, Roqa and Jack, thank you for being really accommodating, easy to work with, and for making me feel super comfortable. And Sam, Andrew and Pippa for the delicious food photography.

Thanks to Luke, my agent, for being so supportive, believing in me and putting 100 per cent into everything. Thanks to my best friend, Georgia, for always being so supportive.

My mum Colette has been there for me throughout all my struggles. She's worked so hard her whole life, and taught me how to work hard, too. Thanks for everything, Mum.

Finally, thank you so much to all the Instagram community and my followers. I really wouldn't be here if it wasn't for you all!

Happier, Healthier, Tastier!